EMOTIONS IN PERSONALITY DISORDERS

EMOTIONS IN PERSONALITY DISORDERS

Edited by
The Guilford Press

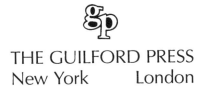

THE GUILFORD PRESS
New York   London

Copyright ©2025 The Guilford Press
A Division of Guilford Publications, Inc.
www.guilford.com

All rights reserved

Printed in the United States of America

This book is printed on acid-free paper.

Last digit is print number: 9 8 7 6 5 4 3 2 1

ISBN: 978-1-4625-5713-4

All articles in this book were previously published in *Journal of Personality Disorders*, Volume 35, Supplement A. ©2021 The Guilford Press.

Preface

This volume presents research into emotions and personality disorders, with a number of chapters focusing on borderline personality disorder (BPD), with its extreme mood swings and labile emotions. All work is current, and represents premier research selected from the *Journal of Personality Disorders*.

Topics are discussed in the broad framework of how emotions—and which emotions—can significantly distinguish among groups to sharpen the therapeutic strategies offered. A range of clinical experts examine emotions such as fearlessness and subjective fear, emotional dysregulation, and shame.

Clinical research delves into treatment method successes as well as possible predictors of behavior. Further research strives to untangle why depression and personality disorder, especially BPD, are so often comorbid, and how emotions like shame, which is a core feature of BPD, shape behavior.

This volume also presents work focusing on dialectical behavior therapy (DBT) and problem-solving techniques in achieving emotional stability; on how beliefs can influence behavior—for the positive as well as the negative; and on how childhood emotional adversity can help predict BPD.

Emotions in Personality Disorders serves as a foundational resource of research on the interactions of emotions and behaviors, prediction, and therapeutic strategies—all through the lens of personality disorders.

Contents

Preface   v

Change of Emotional Experience in Major Depression and Borderline   1
Personality Disorder During Psychotherapy: Associations with
Depression Severity and Personality Functioning
    Ulrike Dinger, DSc, MD, Magdalena Fuchs, MSc, Johanna Köhling, PhD,
    Henning Schauenburg, MD, and Johannes C. Ehrenthal, PhD

Exploring the Effectiveness of Dialectical Behavior Therapy versus   21
Systems Training for Emotional Predictability and Problem Solving
in a Sample of Patients with Borderline Personality Disorder
    Verónica Guillén Botella, PhD, Azucena García-Palacios, PhD,
    Sara Bolo Miñana, MClinPsych, Rosa Baños, PhD,
    Cristina Botella, PhD, and José Heliodoro Marco, PhD

Maladaptive Fearlessness: An Examination of the Association   39
between Subjective Fear Experience and Antisocial Behaviors
Linked with Callous Unemotional Traits
    Elise M. Cardinale, PhD, Rebecca M. Ryan, PhD,
    and Abigail A. Marsh, PhD

Beliefs About Emotion Shift Dynamically Alongside Momentary Affect   57
    Jennifer C. Veilleux, PhD, Elise A. Warner, MSW,
    Danielle E. Baker, MA, and Kaitlyn D. Chamberlain, MA

Emotional Dysregulation and Childhood Adversity in Borderline   88
Personality Disorder
    Emily R. Edwards, PhD, Nina L. J. Rose, MA, Molly Gromatsky, PhD,
    Abigail Feinberg, BA, David Kimhy, PhD, John T. Doucette, PhD,
    Marianne Goodman, MD, Margaret M. McClure, PhD,
    M. Mercedes Perez-Rodriguez, MD, PhD, Antonia S. New, MD,
    and Erin A. Hazlett, PhD

Shame in Borderline Personality Disorder: Meta-Analysis   106
    Tzipi Buchman-Wildbaum, MA, Zsolt Unoka, MD, PhD,
    Robert Dudas, MD, PhD, Gabriella Vizin, PhD,
    Zsolt Demetrovics, PhD, and Mara J. Richman, PhD

Change of Emotional Experience in Major Depression and Borderline Personality Disorder During Psychotherapy: Associations with Depression Severity and Personality Functioning

Ulrike Dinger, DSc, MD, Magdalena Fuchs, MSc, Johanna Köhling, PhD, Henning Schauenburg, MD, and Johannes C. Ehrenthal, PhD

> This study examines emotional experience in major depressive disorder (MDD) with and without comorbid borderline personality disorder (BPD). It investigates if depression severity or personality functioning mediates group differences and which aspects of emotional experience change during psychotherapy. The emotional experience of MDD-BPD patients ($n = 44$) was compared to MDD-only patients ($n = 35$) before and after multimodal short-term psychotherapy. Emotions were classified based on valence and an active/passive polarity. MDD-BPD patients exhibited more active-negative emotions. This group difference was mediated by the level of personality functioning, but not by depression severity. Although passive-negative emotions decreased and positive emotions increased during therapy, there was no significant change in active-negative emotions. The two patient groups did not significantly differ in the change of emotional experience. Lower levels of personality functioning in depressed patients with BPD are associated with a broader spectrum of negative emotions, specifically more active-negative emotions.
>
> *Keywords*: major depression, borderline personality disorder, emotional experience, psychotherapy

Emotions are highly relevant for psychopathology and psychotherapy. They help to appraise oneself and the environment and guide social interactions. Because of their key importance for self-regulation and well-being, disturbances in emotional experiencing are central for the description and phenomenology of psychopathology. The improvement of emotional suffering is an important goal for psychotherapy. The current study seeks to examine differences in the

---

From Center for Psychosocial Medicine, Heidelberg University Hospital.

Ulrike Dinger and Magdalena Fuchs contributed equally to this article.

Address correspondence to Ulrike Dinger, Center for Psychosocial Medicine, Heidelberg University Hospital, Thibautstr. 4, 69115 Heidelberg, Germany. E-mail: ulrike.dinger@med.uni-heidelberg.de

---

Originally published in the *Journal of Personality Disorders*, Volume 35, Supplement A. ©2021 The Guilford Press.

emotional experience as a potential marker for the differentiation between depressed patients with and without borderline personality disorder (BPD) and the change in emotional experience before and after psychotherapy for the two patient groups.

A POLAR CLASSIFICATION OF EMOTIONS

In order to describe patients' emotional experiencing, emotions may be organized according to different classification systems. Most approaches include *valence*, that is, a distinction between positive and negative emotions (e.g., Bradley & Lang, 1994). A second dimension that has been proposed is *arousal* (e.g., Thayer, 1989). High arousal implies physiological activation and preparation for action, while low-arousal emotions tend to decrease activation and suppress actions. The circumplex model of affect integrates the dimensions of valence and arousal (Posner, Russell, & Peterson, 2005).

Other theoretical approaches focus on the directedness of emotions instead of the physiological activation. Dahl (1995) suggested a classification in which emotions are primarily divided into *self*-directed versus *other*-directed (e.g., despair vs. hate). In a second step, Dahl (1995) proposed to cluster emotions according to valence and locus of control. *Active* emotions imply that the subject can exert influence. They are turned outward and often involve aggressive impulses. The reverse is true for *passive* emotions, which refer to situations where a person is not in control (e.g., sadness, anxiety). These emotions are turned inward and can lead to withdrawal. In most cases, active emotions overlap with other-directed emotions because they often relate to another person or an object. Exceptions are irritability (turned outward, but not aiming at an object) or fear (may be connected to another person). The dimension of active and passive also bears some resemblance to the circumplex model because active emotions tend to go hand in hand with high physiological arousal, and passive emotions are likely to be low-arousal emotions. In an attempt to incorporate these different theoretical considerations on emotional experiencing, Benecke, Vogt, Bock, Koschier, and Peham (2008) developed an integrative model for the assessment of emotional experience in clinical samples. Using a self-report, they identified three main factors: *active-negative*, *passive-negative*, and *positive* in accordance with the dimensions of valence and locus of control.

EMOTIONAL EXPERIENCE IN MAJOR DEPRESSION AND BORDERLINE PERSONALITY DISORDER

Major depressive disorder (MDD) and BPD are two common mental disorders that have been repeatedly compared for their presumably different profiles of emotional experience. Broadly speaking, MDD is characterized by deficient positive affect on the one hand, and intensified negative affect on the other. On a more detailed level, certain emotions are particularly relevant to the experience of major depression. *Sadness* belongs to the core emotions that contribute to the experience of anhedonia and depressive mood (e.g., Leventhal, 2008). Feelings of *guilt* and *shame* are also often elevated in patients with depression (e.g., Kim, Thibodeau, & Jorgensen, 2011), and guilt is included as a symptom in several diagnostic instruments, for example, in the Beck Depression Inventory (BDI; Beck, Steer, & Brown, 1996) and the Hamilton Rating Scale for Depression (HRSD; Hamilton, 1960). Research on emotional reactivity indicates a generally reduced responsiveness in depressed individuals, which is true for both positive and negative events (for a review, see Bylsma, Morris, & Rottenberg, 2008). This bears upon another component of the emotional experience in depression: feelings of *numbness*, or the "feeling of not feeling." Depressed patients often describe themselves as empty, numb, or cut off from the world. In this state of reduced or even absent affectivity, life seems to have lost its meaning. As a consequence, depressed patients feel passive, lifeless, and powerless. Taken together, characteristic emotions in MDD are predominantly passive-negative and turned against the self. At the same time, factors such as anger, aggression, irritability, and hostility are common and associated with a worse long-term course in individuals with depression, including chronicity, self-harm, or suicide (e.g., Dumais et al., 2005; Judd, Schettler, Coryell, Akiskal, & Fiedorowicz, 2013). Both aspects of depressive experiences have been formulated in very early writings on the disorders already (Freud, 1917), and they build a bridge toward the understanding of personality-related symptom profiles, for example in comorbid BPD.

Many conceptualizations of BPD view intense and dysregulated negative emotions as a core feature of this disorder (e.g., Linehan, 1993; Zanarini & Frankenburg, 2007). Similar to patients with depression, BPD patients often experience dysphoric states, including passive-negative emotions such as shame, emptiness, and strong feelings of hopelessness (Silk, 2010). In this regard, the emotional experience of BPD patients can overlap with MDD. However, there are a number of other emotions that may be more specific to BPD. Compared to patients with higher levels of personality functioning and to nonclinical control groups, BPD patients seem to be prone to experience more active-negative emotions. A recent systematic review identified higher *anger* and *hostility* in depressed patients with comorbid BPD compared to MDD-only patients (Köhling, Ehrenthal, Levy, Schauenburg, & Dinger, 2015). Single studies showed elevated *disgust* in BPD patients (e.g., Schienle, Haas-Krammer, Schöggl, Kapfhammer, & Ille, 2013), increased *anger* and *fear* (e.g., Leichsenring, 2004), and higher levels of *impulsivity* (e.g., Fertuck et al., 2006). Previous work by Westen et al. (1992) provided further evidence that *emptiness* and *loneliness* are particularly relevant in borderline depression, which is closely tied to fears of abandonment.

In summary, the emotional profile of patients with BPD seems to include a broad spectrum of negative affects. While emotions in patients with MDD are more homogeneous and mainly include passive-negative emotions, BPD patients exhibit more, often conflicting negative emotions, such as anger and sadness. Previous findings further suggest that even currently depressed BPD patients experience more diverse negative affects that do not correspond with the restricted emotional experience that is typical for MDD-only patients.

DIMENSIONAL MODELS OF PERSONALITY FUNCTIONING AND EMOTIONAL EXPERIENCING

A key challenge to the comparison of emotional experiencing between mental disorders comes from the heterogeneity of the diagnostic categories and a considerable range of severity within the different diagnostic categories (e.g., Ehrenthal, Levy, Scott, & Granger, 2018). Proposals from *DSM-5* and ICD-11 task forces suggest incorporating a dimensional rating of personality dysfunction for the diagnosis of personality disorder (PD) (Bender, Morey, & Skodol, 2011; Tyrer et al., 2011) into formal diagnostic procedures. For example, the *DSM-5* Levels of Personality Functioning Scale (LPFS) covers an individual's functioning in the realms of the self and the interpersonal domain (Morey, 2017). Research evidence suggests the assumption of a general severity factor in PDs and supports the model's usefulness for research and practice (e.g., Waugh et al., 2017; Zimmermann, Böhnke, et al., 2015). A similar approach is the Levels of Structural Integration Axis of the Operationalized Psychodynamic Diagnosis system (OPD-LSIA; Taskforce OPD, 2008). It is related to LPFS ratings by expert opinion as well as ratings by untrained students (Zimmermann et al., 2012, 2014).

The emotional experience is included in most approaches to measure levels of personality functioning from slightly varying perspectives. For example, the LPFS summarizes information regarding the ability to experience and regulate emotions within the realm of "identity." The OPD-LSIA addresses the experience of emotions via the subscales experiencing affect, affect differentiation, affect tolerance, and communication of affect. For the OPD-LSIA, studies with expert ratings of emotional facial expressions suggest that higher personality dysfunction is associated with more negative facial expression toward an interaction partner (e.g., more disgust; Bock, Huber, & Benecke, 2016; Peham et al., 2015). Despite the inclusion of some aspects of emotional experience into measures of personality functioning, less is known about the association of levels of personality functioning (including the ability to regulate emotions) with the "content" of emotional experiencing. However, the discrete emotions that are associated with specific clinical disorders continue to be relevant for their diagnosis and treatment. At the same time, the previously described differences in emotional experience between depressed patients with and without comorbid BPD remain poorly understood. The dimensional perspective on personality functioning as a potential mediator variable for these group differences fills a current knowledge gap, because deficits in personality functioning (e.g., lower abilities for affect differentiation and tolerance) may explain why depressed BPD patients experience a range of diverse and sometimes conflicting negative emotions.

STABILITY AND CHANGE OF EMOTIONAL EXPERIENCING IN MDD AND BPD

Emotional experience varies over time. In addition to stable between-person differences (trait-component), affects fluctuate within persons (state-component).

Findings of more average negative emotions in ecological momentary assessment (EMA) studies indicate an elevated negative affect trait in depression and BPD compared to nonclinical controls (e.g., Ebner-Priemer & Trull, 2009). Furthermore, personality traits and personality dysfunction are associated with the temporal stability of emotional experience and related outcome variables in nonclinical groups as well as in patients with depression and BPD (e.g., Hepp, Carpenter, Lane, & Trull, 2016; Miller, Vachon & Lynham, 2009; Roche, 2018), suggesting that they may contribute to the understanding of emotion change over and above diagnostic categories. This is even more important because comparisons of affective instability between clinical groups are inconclusive (e.g., Santangelo et al., 2014). Depressed and BPD samples reported similar levels of affective instability in two EMA studies, but they showed slightly different patterns of reactivity to specific events (Hepp et al., 2016; Köhling et al., 2016). Taken together, EMA studies suggest that personality dysfunction may be relevant for emotion change.

Despite the acknowledgment that emotions are central to the psychotherapeutic treatment of mental disorders (e.g., L. S. Greenberg, 2004; Samoilov & Goldfried, 2000), there is a surprising lack of studies that examine the effect of psychotherapy on patients' emotional experience. Although previous studies have addressed change in emotion regulation strategies (e.g., Berking et al., 2008), or expert ratings of emotion expression (e.g., Leising, Grande, & Faber, 2010), changes in the discrete emotions subjectively experienced by patients before and after psychotherapy have rarely been studied, although the type of affects that need to be regulated (i.e., the content of emotional experiencing) appears highly relevant.

Some subsets of emotions have been implicitly considered as components of broader scales. This is evident in analyses of treatment efficacy for both MDD and BPD, because depression rating scales that are typically used to assess treatment efficacy include certain depression-associated emotions such as anxiety, guilt, sadness, and hopelessness. Therefore, a reduction in overall depression severity implicitly indicates a likely decrease in these depression-associated passive-negative emotions. Previous meta-analyses show that depressed patients score significantly lower on depression scales after psychotherapy (e.g., Barth et al., 2013), indicating that the negative depression-associated emotions decrease with treatment. Instruments for borderline-typical symptomatology also cover some emotions. The Borderline Symptom List (BSL; Bohus et al., 2001) assesses, among other items, loneliness, anger/hostility, and dysphoria. Using the BSL or similar scales, previous meta-analyses have shown that different psychotherapeutic approaches successfully reduce emotional suffering in BPD patients (e.g., Cristea et al., 2017). Nevertheless, specific emotions have only been investigated as a partial aspect of overall symptomatology and treatment outcome. In addition, it is currently unclear if emotions change in a similar way for different clinical groups, and whether or not this change pattern is associated with personality dysfunction. Taking into account the EMA findings from patients' daily life as well as previous psychotherapy outcome findings (e.g., Newton-Howes et al., 2014), personality dysfunction appears as a potential predictor for emotion change as an outcome variable during therapy. To the best of our knowledge, the current study is the first that explicitly examines the change of a broad subset of clinically relevant emotions over the course of a psychotherapeutic intervention for depressed patients with and without comorbid BPD.

AIMS OF THE CURRENT STUDY

The aims of the present study were threefold. First, we examined whether depressed patients with comorbid BPD can be differentiated from depressed patients without BPD by their emotional experience. Second, we aimed to examine whether the expected group differences are mediated by depression severity and/or the level of personality functioning. Third, we asked how the subjective emotional experience changes during an intensive, individually tailored short-time psychotherapy program in the two groups. To do so, we assessed patients' emotions before and after an inpatient multimodal psychotherapy program. We chose to examine women only, because gender is known to influence emotional processing (e.g., Bradley, Codispoti, Sabatinelli, & Lang, 2001) and the majority of patients in both diagnostic groups are women. We expected that MDD-BPD patients would experience more active-negative emotions before the start of treatment, but that there would be no differences in passive-negative or positive emotions between the two groups. We further expected that level of personality functioning and depression severity would mediate the group differences on emotional experience and their change during treatment. Because depressed patients with BPD are usually less responsive to treatment (e.g., M. D. Greenberg, Craighead, Evans, & Craighead, 1995; Unger, Hoffmann, Köhler, Mackert, & Fydrich, 2013), we hypothesized that their emotional experience would improve less during treatment.

METHODS

Participants

The study included 80 adult female inpatients[1] treated at the Department of General Internal Medicine and Psychosomatics, Heidelberg University Hospital, in Germany. All patients met *DSM-IV* (American Psychiatric Association, 2000) diagnostic criteria for current MDD. Forty-four of them also met *DSM-IV* criteria for either full ($n = 39$) or subthreshold ($n = 5$) BPD and were assigned to the MDD-BPD group. The remaining 36 patients did not meet the criteria for any personality disorder. Exclusion criteria were neurological disorders, psychotic disorders, substance dependence with ongoing consumption, and acute suicidality. For the MDD-only group, we excluded patients with any personality disorder. Table 1 shows the demographic and clinical characteristics of the study sample. The groups did not differ in age or current psychotropic medication. Patients in the MDD-BPD group had a higher

---

1. Originally, the sample consisted of 81 recruited participants, but one of them was excluded due to missing data in the Emotional Experience and Emotion Regulation Scale.

TABLE 1. Sample Characteristics and Pre- and Posttreatment Comparisons of Emotions

	MDD-only (n = 36/32)	Mdd+BPD (n = 44/36)	Difference test
Age: M (SD))	28.9 (8.4)	25.8 (7.0)	$t(78) = -1.8, p = .071$
Psychotropic medication: N (%)	16 (44.4)	21 (47.7)	$\chi^2(1) = .027, p = .870$
Number of diagnoses Axis 1: M (SD)	2.2 (1.1)	4.0 (1.5)	$t(78) = 5.90, p < .001$
Affective disorders: N (%)	36 (100.0)	44 (100.0)	
Anxiety disorders: N (%)	10 (27.8)	26 (59.1)	
Somatoform disorders: N (%)	3 (8.3)	2 (4.5)	
Eating disorders: N (%)	6 (16.7)	6 (13.6)	
Substance-related disorders: N (%)	0 (0.0)	4 (9.1)	
Number of diagnoses Axis 2: M (SD)	0 (0.0)	1.7 (0.8)	$t(78) = 12.16, p < .001$
Borderline PD: n (%)	0 (0.0)	39 (88.6)	
Subthreshold BPD: n (%)	0 (0.0)	5 (11.4)	
Avoidant PD: n (%)	0 (0.0)	10 (22.7)	
Dependent PD: n (%)	0 (0.0)	1 (2.3)	
Depressive PD: n (%)	0 (0.0)	10 (22.7)	
Depression Severity			
HRSD: M (SD)	19.4 (5.2)	22.4 (5.5)	$t(78) = 2.54, p = .013$
BDI-II Pretherapy: M (SD)	27.6 (8.8)	33.6 (10.7)	$t(78) = 2.72, p = .008$
BDI-II Posttherapy: M (SD)	16.4 (10.7)	27.1 (14.5)	$t(66) = 3.43, p = .001$
OPD-SQ: M (SD)	1.9 (0.4)	2.5 (0.5)	$t(78) = 5.29, p < .001$
Emotions Pretherapy			
Active-negative: M (SD)	2.02 (1.10)	2.75 (1.20)	$t(78) = 2.84, p = .006*$
Passive-negative: M (SD)	3.23 (1.24)	3.65 (1.11)	$t(78) = 1.58, p = .118$
Positive: M (SD)	1.46 (0.59)	1.19 (0.68)	$t(78) = -1.59, p = .117$
Emotions Posttherapy			
Active-negative: M (SD)	1.76 (1.20)	2.71 (1.52)	$t(66) = 2.82, p = .006*$
Passive-negative: M (SD)	2.48 (1.46)	3.37 (1.34)	$t(66) = 2.62, p = .011*$
Positive: M (SD)	2.26 (1.19)	1.76 (1.04)	$t(66) = -1.86, p = .068$

Note. M = Mean, SD = Standard Deviation, HRSD = Hamilton Rating Scale for Depression, OPD-SQ = Operationalized Psychodynamic Diagnosis Structure Questionnaire. Ns were smaller posttreatment due to dropouts.
*Bonferroni corrected alpha level of $p < .017$, all two-tailed t tests.

number of both Axis I and Axis II disorders. Due to treatment dropouts during therapy, the sample size was reduced to 68 subjects at the posttreatment assessment (three MDD-only dropouts, nine MDD-BPD dropouts).

Procedure

Participants were consecutively recruited following admission to the Department of General Internal Medicine and Psychosomatics, Heidelberg University Hospital. Those who gave written informed consent received structured diagnostic interviews, were rated on the HRSD by two independent observers, and filled out questionnaires at admission and discharge. The study was approved by the local institutional review board of the Medical Faculty, Heidelberg University.

Patients were treated in one of two inpatient psychotherapy units within the same hospital. All patients received psychodynamic individual psychotherapy, psychodynamic group therapy, one or more nonverbal group therapies (art, concentrated-movement, and/or music therapy), and social competence trainings. In addition, some patients received a stabilization group aimed at the establishment of better emotion regulation skills, some patients participated in a mindfulness group, and some took part in a relaxation group. For each patient, an individual psychotherapeutic focus was defined with the goal of tailoring the psychotherapy program to the level of personality functioning and the assumed psychodynamics underlying the patient's mental health symptoms. Treatment duration was 8–10 weeks. The majority of patients were treated as inpatients. However, six participants in the MDD-only group were day-clinic patients because one of the units combines an inpatient with a day-clinic setting (e.g., Dinger et al., 2014). The inpatient and day-clinic units are open facilities, all patients were treated voluntarily in their respective setting, and they were free to leave the unit at any point during treatment.

Measures

DSM-IV Diagnoses. The Structured Clinical Interviews for *DSM-IV* Axis I and Axis II Disorders (SCID-I and SCID-II; First, Gibbon, Spitzer, Williams, & Benjamin, 1997; First, Spitzer, Gibbon, & Williams, 1997) were used to assess psychiatric disorders according to *DSM-IV*. Both interviews are well established and frequently used diagnostic instruments that have shown sufficient to good interrater reliability (κs > .70 and κs > .65, respectively, First, Gibbon, et al., 1997; First, Spitzer, et al., 1997).[2]

Emotional Experience. The Emotional Experience and Emotion Regulation Scale (EER; Benecke et al., 2008) was used for the assessment of emotions. It consists of two parts; only the first part (with 59 items on emotional experience) was administered in this study. The scale includes 20 subscales for specific emotions with three items each.[3] Participants are asked to rate how intensely they experienced a feeling during the past 7 days on a 7-point scale ranging from 0 (*not at all*) to 6 (*extremely*). The 20 subscales are grouped into three main scales based on a second-order factor analysis: *active-negative* emotions (anger, contempt, disgust, envy/jealousy, impulsivity, irritability, uninhibitedness, uncontrollability), *passive-negative* emotions (diffuse anxiety,

---

2. In the current study, the structured diagnostic interviews were conducted by a PhD student in clinical psychology, who had finished previous training in SCID-I and SCID-II interviews and received continuous supervision throughout this study. Because only one person conducted the interview, no interrater reliability is available here.
3. The scale envy/jealousy is an exception and includes only two items.

fear, guilt, helplessness, lifelessness, loneliness, sadness, shame), and *positive* emotions (interest, joy, love/affection, surprise). In the current study, the three second-order emotion scales were used, each with high internal reliability (Cronbach's αs of .92, .94, and .81 for active-negative, passive-negative, and positive, respectively).

Depression Severity. The HRSD (Hamilton, 1960) was used to assess depression severity from the perspective of an independent observer. The HRSD is an expert rating scale designed to measure severity of depression over the previous week. In this study, two master's-level psychologists independently rated the 17-item version based on a brief standardized interview. Interrater reliability was excellent, with intraclass correlation (ICC) (2, 2) = .86. The mean value of the two ratings was used for all subsequent analyses.

The BDI-II (Beck et al., 1996) was used to assess depression severity by patient self-report. The BDI-II measures cognitive and somatic-affective symptoms of depression with 21 items. Patients are asked to rate the severity of each symptom on a 4-point scale; depression severity is calculated as the sum score from all items. In addition to the global sum score, cognitive and somatic-affective subscales have been proposed (Beck et al., 1996). The BDI-II is a frequently used, reliable measure of depressive symptoms. Cronbach's α was .87 for the global sum score in the current sample at intake.

Personality Functioning. The OPD-SQ (Ehrenthal et al., 2012) is a self-report on personality functioning in accordance with the OPD-LSIA (OPD Taskforce, 2008). It consists of eight subscales and 95 items rated on a 5-point scale. An overall severity index is calculated by the mean of the subscales, with higher scores indicating higher impairment. The OPD-SQ correlates with expert-ratings of the OPD-LSIA, other measures of personality and attachment, as well as the number of *DSM-IV* PD diagnoses (Dinger, et al., 2014), and captures the general features of personality disorders (Zimmermann, Dahlbender et al., 2015). In this study, the OPD-SQ overall severity index had excellent internal consistency (Cronbach's α = .94).

Data Analysis

We compared depression severity, level of personality functioning, and emotional experience with t tests for independent groups. For the test of Hypothesis 1 (group difference in emotional experience), the tests of the three main EER scales were Bonferroni-corrected for multiple comparisons (α = 0.05/3). Group differences for single emotions were further explored via non-Bonferroni–corrected comparisons.

Given the nested structure of the pre-post data, multilevel modeling (Raudenbush & Bryk, 2002) was used to identify relevant predictors of emotions at the two assessments for the tests of Hypothesis 2 (mediation of group differences) and Hypothesis 3 (pre-post change). We constructed a set of four different multilevel regression models for each of the three dependent variables (active-negative, active-passive and positive emotions).[4] All models included time (pre- vs. posttherapy) as a predictor in addition to the intercept, and a random effect of subjects in order to account for within-subject variation in emotional experience. Model I further included group (MDD-only vs. MDD-BPD), and the Time × Group interaction as fixed effects and examined whether a comorbid BPD had an effect on the emotion scales or their change during treatment. Model II included the same predictors as Model I plus the HRSD score and its interaction with time in order to examine the influence of depression severity on emotional experience. Model III replaced the HRSD by the OPD-SQ and tested the effect of personality functioning on emotional experience. Finally, Model IV included all previous predictors on the intercept in order to examine the relative influence of each predictor while controlling for the other. The Bayesian Information Criterion (BIC) was chosen as a descriptive fit index.[5] These statistical analyses were performed using R (open source, www.r-project.org, version 3.2.2). In case of indications for a possible mediation of the group effect by either depression severity and/or personality functioning in the MLMs, we planned to conduct a separate mediation analysis with the R package by Tingley, Yamamoto, Hirose, Keele, and Imai (2014).

RESULTS

Group Comparisons Pre- and Posttherapy

As shown in Table 1, patients with BPD were characterized by higher depression severity compared to patients with MDD only. They also exhibited higher impairment in personality functioning as measured by the OPD-SQ. The Bonferroni-corrected group comparisons of the EER main scales revealed significant differences in the experience of active-negative emotions. The MDD-BPD group scored higher on the active-negative scale than the MDD-only group, both pre- and posttreatment. Neither the passive-negative nor the positive scale differed between the two groups before treatment. However, BPD patients reported significantly higher passive-negative emotions after therapy (see Figure 1).

Further exploratory (non-Bonferroni–corrected) t tests of the EER active-negative subscale indicated that the MDD-BPD group experienced more *disgust* [$t(78) = 3.94, p < .01$, Cohen's $d = 0.89$], *contempt* [$t(77) = 3.18, p < .01$, Cohen's $d = 0.72$], *impulsivity* [$t(78) = 2.90, p < .01$, Cohen's $d = 0.66$], and *uninhibitedness* [$t(78) = 2.82, p < .01$, Cohen's $d = 0.64$] before treatment. These differences remained stable after treatment [disgust: $t(66) = 3.23, p < .01$,

---

4. Before deciding on the final predictors of the models, we examined whether the effects on emotion scales were influenced by the small number of day-clinic patients in the MDD-only group or the number of subthreshold patients in the BPS group. This was not the case, so we did not include those variables in the final model.
5. Because the models were not nested, it was not possible to compare their fit to the data based on a significance test.

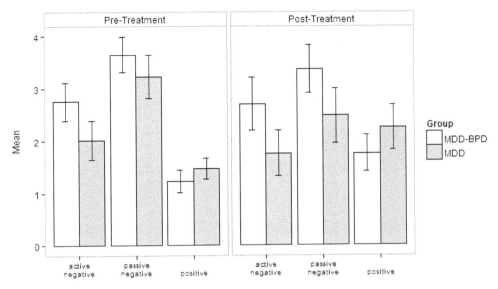

FIGURE 1. Emotion scale scores by diagnostic group with 95% confidence intervals. MDD = major depressive disorder; BPD = borderline personality disorder.

Cohen's $d = 0.79$; contempt: $t(66) = 3.17, p < .01$, Cohen's $d = 0.78$; impulsivity: $t(66) = 2.19, p = .032$, Cohen's $d = 0.54$; uninhibitedness: $t(66) = 2.23$, $p = .029$, Cohen's $d = 0.55$]. Contrary to expectations, anger did not significantly differ between the groups [pre: $t(78) = 1.45, p = .15$, Cohen's $d = 0.33$]; post: $t(66) = 1.77, p = .09$, Cohen's $d = 0.44$]. A further examination of *loneliness* showed higher levels in the MDD-BPD group [pre: $(t(78) = 2.97, p < .01$, Cohen's $d = 0.67$; post: $(t(66) = 2.70, p < .01$, Cohen's $d = 0.66$].

Prediction of Emotional Experience

A series of four multilevel models was repeated for each EER scale as dependent variable (see Table 2). Model I served to analyze whether a comorbid BPD was associated with experience of emotions and/or change during treatment. Being in the BPD group corresponded with more active-negative emotions, but had no effect on the other two emotion scales. The effect of time was different for the three emotion scales. During treatment, participants' reports of passive-negative emotions decreased, while positive emotions increased. Time had no effect on active-negative emotions. The interaction between time and group was not significant for any of the three emotion scales, which indicates that the slope of change did not differ significantly between the two groups.

To examine the influence of initial depression severity, Model II included the HRSD and its interaction with time. The effects of time and group were similar to those of Model I. In addition, more severely depressed patients experienced more passive-negative emotions. However, the HRSD predicted neither the active-negative nor the positive emotions. The interaction between time and the HRSD was not significant for any of the emotion scales.

TABLE 2. Four Multilevel Models for Three Emotion Scales

	Active Negative				Passive Negative				Positive			
	Model I	Model II	Model III	Model IV	Model I	Model II	Model III	Model IV	Model I	Model II	Model III	Model IV
Intercept	2.79***	2.72***	2.5***	2.44***	3.77***	3.67***	3.49***	3.37***	1.17***	1.14***	1.23***	1.25***
Time	−0.08	−0.18	−0.18	−0.18	−0.4*	−0.58***	−0.58***	−0.58***	0.59***	0.71***	0.72***	0.71***
Group (MDD)	−0.75*	−0.61*	−0.14	−0.00	−0.51	−0.3	0.09	0.34	0.25	0.3	0.12	0.07
HRSD	—	0.26	—	0.27	—	0.47**	—	—	—	−0.07	—	−0.09
OPD-SQ	—	—	0.59**	0.56***	—	—	0.58***	0.49***	—	—	−0.18	−0.21
Time × Group	−0.2	—	—	—	−0.38	—	—	0.60***	0.26	—	—	—
Time × HRSD	—	0.15	—	—	—	0.18	—	—	—	−0.1	—	—
Time × OPD-SF	—	—	0.04	—	—	—	0.2	—	—	—	−0.08	—
BIC	433.87	432.89	426.39	422.74	450.96	439.96	438.13	424.66	367.01	370.82	368.62	368.13

Note. HRSD = Hamilton Rating Scale for Depression; OPD-SQ = Operationalized Psychodynamic Diagnosis-Structure Questionnaire; BIC = Bayesian Information Criterion. Standardized β coefficients. *$p < .05$. **$p < .01$. ***$p < .001$.

Model III examined the effect of personality functioning on emotional experience. Thus, the HRSD was replaced by the OPD-SQ. Again, change during therapy (time) showed the same pattern as before, but the effect of group on the active-negative emotions was no longer significant with the inclusion of the OPD-SQ. Patients with lower levels of personality functioning experienced both more passive-negative and more active-negative emotions. The OPD-SQ did not have an effect on the positive emotions. The interaction between time and OPD-SQ was not significant for any emotion scale.

Finally, Model IV compared the relative influence of all predictors examined so far. Because none of the predictors had previously been associated with the rate of change, all interactions with time were dropped from the model. As in Models I–III, participants' reports of passive-negative emotions decreased from pre- to posttreatment, while their reports of positive emotions increased, and there was no change in active-negative emotions. When controlling for the other predictors, group did not significantly predict any one of the three emotion scales. Again, depression severity predicted more passive-negative emotions, but neither the active-negative nor the positive emotions. The level of personality functioning predicted both the active- and passive-negative emotions, but not the positive emotions.

In order to understand the relative influence of the variables of interest, particularly depression severity and personality functioning, the chosen models were not nested within one another. Although a direct comparison of the models' explanatory power was not possible, we report the BIC for descriptive purposes.

Mediation Analysis

Patients in the MDD-BPD group experienced more active-negative emotions than MDD-only patients, but this effect disappeared when the OPD-SQ was entered into the model. The OPD-SQ was the only variable whose inclusion into the model affected the group effect on one of the emotion scales. Thus, we conducted a mediation analysis considering the impact of group and OPD-SQ on the active-negative scale. For this analysis, we used Imai et al.'s (2010) general approach to causal mediation analysis. The total effect of group on active-negative emotions was −.846 (95% CI [−1.247, −0.443], $p < .001$). However, 82.5% of the total effect was mediated by OPD-SQ ($p < .001$). Controlling for this indirect effect, the direct effect of group became insignificant (−.150, 95% CI [−0.643, −0.319], $p = .56$).

DISCUSSION

Due to the high co-occurrence of depressive disorders and BPD together with a considerable symptom overlap, the emotional experience of depressed patients with and without comorbid BPD continues to be an important object of investigation. Congruent with our hypotheses, the current findings revealed that depressed patients with BPD experienced active-negative emotions more intensely than those without BPD. Even after treatment, this group effect remained significant, suggesting a robust distinction. This pattern replicates findings that intense active-negative emotions, which involve strong or even uncontrollable impulses for action, are specific features of BPD patients. A number of previous studies showed that depressed patients with comorbid BPD report higher levels of anger, hostility, and impulsivity than MDD-only patients (Köhling et al., 2015). Interestingly, the exploratory analysis of single emotions showed no group difference for anger, while levels of disgust, contempt, impulsivity, and uninhibitedness were higher in the MDD-BPD group. Despite the nonsignificant group difference for anger, these findings are partially consistent with theoretical approaches that view aggressive and self-destructive affects as a core feature of BPD. According to Perry and Cooper (1985), BPD patients typically have a long-standing sense of rage that often erupts in self-destructive impulses and acts. Similarly, object relations theory emphasizes aggression as a reaction to repeated experiences of pain and frustration as a central characteristic of BPD (Clarkin, Lenzenweger, Yeomans, Levy, & Kernberg, 2007). It has further been argued that the dysphoria in BPD patients stems—at least partially—from their view of themselves as fundamentally bad, guilty, and evil (Gunderson, 2001). Other theorists regard a general emotional dysregulation and extreme negative affectivity as characteristic of BPD (Linehan, 1993; Zanarini & Frankenburg, 2007). This is in line with the fact that the MDD-BPD group in this study reported more impulsivity and uninhibitedness.

The passive-negative emotions of the depressed BPD patients at the start of treatment were not significantly higher than those of the MDD-only group. Among the passive emotions, loneliness was the only one that was rated more intensely by the MDD-BPD group. Although some authors have emphasized the role of loneliness in borderline depression (e.g., Westen et al., 1992), there has been little empirical evidence for this claim so far. However, the current exploratory result is in line with findings from an EMA study where individuals with BPD and a comorbid depression reported lower levels of mood after situations in which they were alone (Köhling et al., 2016). This points to the frequently mentioned difficulties of patients with BPD in building and maintaining stable, harmonious relationships, real ones as well as in the internal, representational world.

In summary, the depressed BPD patients in this study were characterized by a broad spectrum of negative affects. They experienced dysphoric self-directed emotions as well as latent hostile other-directed emotions, whereas in the MDD-only group the passive-negative emotions (e.g., sadness, guilt, or lifelessness) were prevailing.

Mediation of Group Differences

The described group differences in the emotional profile between depressed patients with and without comorbid BPD replicate and extend previous findings. However, the mere description of group differences has only limited value for understanding why the BPD patients experience more active-negative emotions. One hypothesis might be that the difference could be due to a higher depression severity in BPD patients. Congruent with the findings from

Köhling et al.'s (2015) meta-analysis, MDD-BPD patients in this study were rated as more severely depressed than those in the MDD-only group. Also in line with expectations, depression severity predicted the level of passive-negative emotions. However, depression severity did not predict higher levels of active-negative emotions. As a consequence, the broader emotional profile of depressed patients with BPD compared to patients with MDD-only appears to be independent of depression severity.

The level of personality functioning as measured by the OPD-SQ was a significant predictor for the experience of both active- and passive-negative emotions. Furthermore, the mediation analysis showed that the effect of group on active-negative emotions was mediated by the OPD-SQ; that is, the severity of personality dysfunction accounted for the difference in active-negative emotions between the MDD-BPD and the MDD-only groups. In the OPD system, personality functioning is conceptualized as levels of structural integration. These levels are defined via four basic functions: perception of self and objects, regulation of self and relationships, communication with the internal and external worlds, and attachment to internal and external objects (OPD Taskforce, 2008). Lower levels of structural integration manifest themselves, among other aspects, in reduced abilities to understand, regulate, or express emotions and in an intensified negative affect. Thus, the current findings are in line with the OPD model that higher impairment in personality functioning is associated with more diverse and more intense negative emotions. This study adds to the increasing consensus that a dimensional approach to PDs is more accurate, while allowing a differentiated profile diagnosis as a target for psychotherapeutic interventions (Dinger et al., 2014; Trull & Durrett, 2005). The current findings therefore support the importance of a dimensional assessment of personality functioning.

Change of Emotional Profiles over the Course of Treatment

Across patient groups, positive emotions increased from pre- to posttreatment, while passive-negative emotions decreased and there was no change in active-negative emotions. After therapy, patients with BPD reported higher levels of active-negative as well as passive-negative emotions compared to the MDD-only patients. The fact that the passive-negative difference emerged only after treatment might suggest that BPD patients benefit less from treatment. This would have been consistent with previous findings that depression symptoms change slower in BPD (e.g., M. D. Greenberg et al., 1995; Unger et al., 2013). However, the more rigorous test of a systematic difference in the rate of change via multilevel modeling did not support this hypothesis. The Time × Group interaction for passive-negative emotions was not significant ($\beta = 0.38$, $t = 1.36$, $p = .18$), indicating that despite a descriptive trend in the expected direction, the rate of change did not differ significantly between the two groups.

Compared to the literature and our expectations, the MDD-BPD group improved more than anticipated. When speculating about potential explanations, we might focus on the individual therapy and the high clinical experience of psychotherapists with BPD patients on the inpatient units. In line with the OPD system, each patient is treated according to an initial psychodynamic treatment focus. Therapists receive frequent supervision and are specifically trained in OPD-based, structure-oriented therapy, which targets individual deficits in personality functioning (Ehrenthal & Benecke, 2019; Rudolf, 2013). In addition, some elements of the multimodal treatments are tailored to the level of personality functioning (i.e., only patients with deficits in personality functioning participate in a stabilization group, which aims at better self-regulation). Consequently, depressed patients with BPD might have responded comparatively well to treatment. In addition, a stronger regression to the mean effect in the MDD-BPD group may have also contributed to the lack of significantly different rates of change between the two groups. However, given the slight trend in the data, a study with higher statistical power may nevertheless have revealed the expected group difference.

Several explanations are possible for the finding that active-negative emotions did not significantly change during treatment. It could be the case that those emotions are in general more difficult to change, especially within short-term psychotherapy. As pointed out earlier, they involve strong impulses, often arise suddenly and unpredictably, and are thus more difficult to regulate. In addition, it can be argued that the stable level of experienced active-negative emotions in the current study reflects the fact that these emotions belong to the traitlike emotional profile of BPD patients, and that a change of personality pathology requires longer treatment than treatment of depressive symptoms.

Limitations

Despite a large body of literature on the differentiation between depressive disorders and depression in BPD, this is the first study to compare the emotional experience of depressed patients with and without BPD over the course of psychotherapy. A major strength of the current approach was the exploration of a broad set of emotions based on a theoretically sound and empirically tested classification that is particularly suited for clinical contexts. Nevertheless, some limitations need to be acknowledged. First, it is important to note that the present study does not clarify whether BPD patients without a depressive episode experience have equal levels of passive-negative emotions. In order to examine the extent to which emotional experience in the MDD-BPD group was cumulative (i.e., resulting from the two disorders), future studies should include a control group with nondepressed BPD-only patients. Second, the sample size was large enough to test a moderate group difference with sufficient power, but the detection of smaller effects was not adequately powered. Furthermore, the sample was too small to test three-way interactions between time, group, and continuous variables (i.e., HRSD or OPD-SQ) and did not allow inference statistics with Bonferroni correction of the single emotions that were assessed. We therefore focused on the second-order categories of active-negative, passive-negative, and positive emotions. Third, the self-report measure to assess patients' emotional experience may be influenced by recall biases, the immediate affective and cognitive context, or social desirability. For example, the affective instability that is a diagnostic criterion for BPD may cause a differential recall in depressed BPD patients compared to MDD-only patients. More frequent assessments via EMA try to reduce recall biases and have been used for comparisons of BPD patients with other clinical groups such as depressed patients (e.g., Köhling et al., 2016). A fourth limitation lies in the naturalistic study design, which only allowed us to treat the multimodal intervention as a whole "package." As such, we were not able to control for effects of specific interventions, individual patient experiences, or more detailed data on psychotropic drug categories and dosages. This would have been desirable because different medications can influence the processing of emotions. Finally, we chose to examine only female patients because women have a higher prevalence in both disorders, especially in BPD. This decision for greater homogeneity reduces generalizability, which is especially important, because most studies indicate stable gender differences in emotional processing. Women tend to react with more negative valence and greater arousal to aversive stimuli (e.g., Bradley et al., 2001; Gomez, von Gunten, & Danuser, 2013), which is particularly relevant for the study of patients, who can be expected to frequently encounter unpleasant events. It is therefore important to keep in mind that the current findings are limited to female patients.

Summary

The current study showed that depressed patients with BPD can be distinguished from depressed patients without BPD by their emotional experience before and after short-term psychotherapy. Patients with a comorbid BPD had more intense negative emotions and were characterized by a broader spectrum of emotions. Therefore, assessing patients' emotional experience can be helpful for the differential diagnosis of depression.

REFERENCES

American Psychiatric Association. (2000). *Diagnostic and statistical manual of mental disorders* (4th ed., text rev.). Washington, DC: Author.

Barth, J., Munder, T., Gerger, H., Nuesch, E., Trelle, S., Znoj, H., . . . Cuijpers, P. (2013). Comparative efficacy of seven psychotherapeutic interventions for patients with depression: A network meta-analysis. *PLoS Medicine, 10*, e1001454. doi:10.1371/journal.pmed.1001454

Beck, A. T., Steer, R. A., & Brown, G. K. (1996). *Manual for the Beck Depression Inventory-II*. San Antonio, TX: Psychological Corporation.

Bender, D. S., Morey, L. C., & Skodol, A. E. (2011). Toward a model for assessing level of personality functioning in *DSM-5*, part I: A review of theory and methods. *Journal of Personality Assessment, 93*, 332–346. doi:10.1080/00223891.2011.583808

Benecke, C., Vogt, T., Bock, A., Koschier, A., & Peham, D. (2008). Emotionserleben und Emotionsregulation und ihr Zusammenhang mit psychischer Symptomatik [A Self-Report Questionnaire for the Assessment of Emotional Experience and Emotion Regulation]. *Psychotherapie, Psychosomatik, medizinische Psychologie, 58*, 366–370. doi:10.1055/s-2007-986319

Berking, M., Wupperman, P., Reichardt, A., Pejic, T., Dippel, A., & Znoj, H. (2008). Emotion-regulation skills as a treatment target in psychotherapy. *Behaviour Research and Therapy, 46*, 1230–1237. doi:10.1016/j.brat.2008.08.005

Bock, A., Huber, E., & Benecke, C. (2016). Levels of structural integration and facial expressions of negative emotions. *Zeitschrift für Psychosomatische Medizin und Psychotherapie, 62*, 224–238. doi:10.13109/zptm.2016.62.3.224

Bohus, M., Limberger, M. F., Frank, U., Sender, I., Gratwohl, T., & Stieglitz, R. D. (2001). Entwicklung der Borderline-Symptom-Liste [Development of the Borderline-Symptom-List]. *Psychotherapie, Psychosomatik,* medizinische Psychologie, 51, 201–211. doi:10.1055/s-2001-13281

Bradley, M. M., Codispoti, M., Sabatinelli, D., & Lang, P. J. (2001). Emotion and motivation II: Sex differences in picture processing. Emotion, 1, 300–319. doi:10.1037//1528-3542.1.3.300

Bradley, M. M., & Lang, P. J. (1994). Measuring emotion: The self-assessment manikin and the semantic differential. Journal of Behavior Therapy and Experimental Psychiatry, 25, 49–59. doi:10.1016/0005-7916(94)90063-9

Bylsma, L. M., Morris, B. H., & Rottenberg, J. (2008). A meta-analysis of emotional reactivity in major depressive disorder. Clinical Psychology Review, 28, 676–691. doi:10.1016/j.cpr.2007.10.001

Clarkin, J. F., Lenzenweger, M. F., Yeomans, F., Levy, K. N., & Kernberg, O. F. (2007). An object relations model of borderline pathology. Journal of Personality Disorders, 21, 474–499. doi:10.1521/pedi.2007.21.5.474

Cristea, I. A., Gentili, C., Cotet, C. D., Palomba, D., Barbui, C., & Cuijpers, P. (2017). Efficacy of psychotherapies for borderline personality disorder: A systematic review and meta-analysis. JAMA Psychiatry, 74, 319–328. doi:10.1001/jamapsychiatry.2016.4287

Dahl, H. (1995). An information feedback theory of emotions and defenses. In H. Conte & R. Plutchik (Eds.), Ego defenses: Theory and measurement (pp. 98–119). New York, NY: Wiley.

Dinger, U., Klipsch, D., Köhling, J., Ehrenthal, J. C., Nikendei, C., Herzog, W., & Schauenberg, H. (2014). Day-clinic and inpatient psychotherapy for depression (DIP-D): A randomized controlled pilot study in routine clinical care. Psychotherapy and Psychosomatics, 83, 194–195. doi:10.1159/000357437

Dinger, U., Schauenburg, H., Hörz, S., Rentrop, M., Komo-Lang, M., Klinkerfuß, M., . . . Ehrenthal, J. C. (2014). Self-report and observer ratings of personality functioning: A study of the OPD system. Journal of Personality Assessment, 96, 220–225. doi:10.1080/00223891.2013.828065

Dumais, A., Lesage, A. D., Alda, M., Rouleau, G., Dumont, M., Chawky, N., . . . Turecki, G. (2005). Risk factors for suicide completion in major depression: A case-control study of impulsive and aggressive behaviors in men. American Journal of Psychiatry, 162, 2116–2124. doi:10.1176/appi.ajp.162.11.2116

Ebner-Priemer, U. W., & Trull, T. J. (2009). Ecological momentary assessment of mood disorders and mood dysregulation. Psychological Assessment, 21, 463–475. doi:10.1037/a0017075

Ehrenthal, J. C., & Benecke, C. (2019). Tailored treatment planning for individuals with personality disorders: The OPD approach. In U. Kramer (Ed.), Case formulation for personality disorders: Tailoring psychotherapy to the individual client (pp. 291–314). Cambridge, MA: Elsevier.

Ehrenthal, J. C., Dinger, U., Horsch, L., Komo-Lang, M., Klinkerfuss, M., Grande, T., & Schauenburg, H. (2012). The OPD Structure Questionnaire (OPD-SQ): First results on reliability and validity. Psychotherapie, Psychosomatik, medizinische Psychologie, 62, 25–32. doi:10.1055/s-0031-1295481

Ehrenthal, J. C., Levy, K. N., Scott, L. N., & Granger, D. A. (2018). Attachment-related regulatory processes moderate the impact of adverse childhood experiences on stress reaction in borderline personality disorder. Journal of Personality Disorders, 32, 93–114. doi:10.1521/pedi.2018.32.supp.93

Fertuck, E. A., Marsano-Jozefowicz, S., Stanley, B., Tryon, W. W., Oquendo, M., Mann, J. J., & Keilp, J. G. (2006). The impact of borderline personality disorder and anxiety on neuropsychological performance in major depression. Journal of Personality Disorders, 20, 55–70. doi:10.1521/pedi.2006.20.1.55

First, M. B., Gibbon, M., Spitzer, R. L., Williams, J. B. W., & Benjamin, L. S. (1997). Structured Clinical Interview for DSM-IV Axis II Personality Disorders (SCID-II). Washington, DC: American Psychiatric Press.

First, M. B., Spitzer, R. L., Gibbon, M., & Williams, J. B. W. (1997). Structured Clinical Interview for DSM-IV Axis I disorders (SCID-I). New York, NY: Biometric Research Department.

Freud, S. (1917). Trauer und Melancholie [Mourning and Melancholia]. Internationale Zeitschrift für ärztliche Psychoanalyse, 4, 288–301.

Gomez, P., von Gunten, A., & Danuser, B. (2013). Content-specific gender differences in emotion ratings from early to late adulthood. Scandinavian Journal of Psychology, 54, 451–458. doi:10.1111/sjop.12075

Greenberg, L. S. (2004). Emotion-focused therapy. Clinical Psychology & Psychotherapy, 11, 3–16. doi:10.1002/cpp.388

Greenberg, M. D., Craighead, W. E., Evans, D. D., & Craighead, L. W. (1995). An investigation of the effects of comorbid Axis II pathology on outcome of inpatient treatment for unipolar depression. Journal of Psychopathology and Behavioral Assessment, 17, 305–321. doi:10.1007/BF02229053

Gunderson, J. G. (2001). Borderline personality disorder: A clinical guide. Washington, DC: American Psychiatric Publishing.

Hamilton, M. (1960). A rating scale for depression. Journal of Neurology, Neurosurgery, & Psychiatry, 23, 56–62. doi:10.1136/jnnp.23.1.56

Hepp, J., Carpenter, R. W., Lane, S. P., & Trull, T. J. (2016). Momentary symptoms of borderline personality disorder as a product of trait personality and social context. *Personality Disorders: Theory, Research, and Treatment, 7,* 384–393. doi:10.1037/per0000175

Judd, L. L., Schettler, P. J., Coryell, W., Akiskal, H. S., & Fiedorowicz, J. G. (2013). Overt irritability/anger in unipolar major depressive episodes. *JAMA Psychiatry, 70,* 1171–1180. doi:10.1001/jamapsychiatry.2013.1957

Kim, S., Thibodeau, R., & Jorgensen, R. S. (2011). Shame, guilt, and depressive symptoms. *Psychological Bulletin, 137,* 68–96. doi:10.1037/a0021466

Köhling, J., Ehrenthal, J. C., Levy, K. N., Schauenburg, H., & Dinger, U. (2015). Quality and severity of depression in borderline personality disorder: A systematic review and meta-analysis. *Clinical Psychology Review, 37,* 13–25. doi:10.1016/j.cpr.2015.02.002

Köhling, J., Moessner, M., Ehrenthal, J. C., Bauer, S., Cierpka, M., Kämmerer, A., ... Dinger, U. (2016). Affective instability and reactivity in depressed patients with and without borderline pathology. *Journal of Personality Disorders, 30,* 762–775. doi:10.1521/pedi_2015_29_230

Leichsenring, F. (2004). Phänomenologie und Psychodynamik der Affekte bei Borderline-Störungen [Phenomenology and Psychodynamics of Affects in Borderline Personality Disorder]. *Zeitschrift für Psychosomatische Medizin und Psychotherapie, 50,* 253–270. doi:10.2307/23869534

Leising, D., Grande, T., & Faber, R. (2010). A longitudinal study of emotional experience, expressivity, and psychopathology in psychotherapy inpatients and psychologically healthy persons. *Journal of Clinical Psychology, 66,* 1027–1043. doi:10.1002/jclp.20704

Leventhal, A. M. (2008). Sadness, depression, and avoidance behavior. *Behavior Modification, 32,* 759–779. doi:10.1177/0145445508317167

Linehan, M. M. (1993). *Cognitive-behavioral treatment of borderline personality disorder.* New York, NY: Guilford Press.

Miller, D., Vachon, D. D., & Lynam, D. R. (2009). Neuroticism, negative affect, and negative affect instability: Establishing convergent and discriminant validity using ecological momentary assessment. *Personality and Individual Differences, 47,* 873–877. doi:10.1016/j.paid.2009.07.007

Morey, L. C. (2017). Application of the *DSM-5* Level of Personality Functioning Scale by lay raters. *Journal of Personality Disorders, 32,* 709–720. doi:10.1521/pedi_2017_31_305

Newton-Howes, G., Tyrer, P., Johnson, T., Mulder, R., Kool, S., Dekker, J., & Schoevers, R. (2014). Influence of personality on the outcome of treatment in depression: Systematic review and meta-analysis. *Journal of Personality Disorders, 28,* 577–593. doi:10.1521/pedi_2013_27_070

Peham, D., Bock, A. Schiestl, C., Huber, E., Zimmermann, J., Kratzer, D., ... Benecke, C. (2015). Facial affective behavior in mental disorder. *Journal of Nonverbal Behavior, 39,* 371–396. doi:10.1007/s10919-015-0216-6

Perry, J. C., & Cooper, S. H. (1985). Psychodynamics, symptoms, and outcome in borderline and antisocial personality disorders and bipolar type II affective disorder. In T. H. McGlashan (Ed.), *The borderline: Current empirical research* (pp. 21–41). Washington, DC: American Psychiatric Press.

Posner, J., Russell, J. A., & Peterson, B. S. (2005). The circumplex model of affect: An integrative approach to affective neuroscience, cognitive development, and psychopathology. *Development and Psychopathology, 17,* 715–734. doi:10.1017/S0954579405050340

Raudenbush, S. W., & Bryk, A. S. (2002). *Hierarchical linear models: Applications and data analysis methods* (2nd ed.). Thousand Oaks, CA: Sage.

Roche, M. J. (2018). Examining the alternative model for personality disorder in daily life: Evidence for incremental validity. *Personality Disorders: Theory, Research, and Treatment, 9,* 574–583. doi:10.1037/per0000295

Rudolf, G. (2013). *Strukturbezogene Psychotherapie* [Structure-oriented psychotherapy]. Stuttgart, Germany: Schattauer.

Samoilov, A., & Goldfried, M. R. (2000). Role of emotion in cognitive–behavior therapy. *Clinical Psychology: Science and Practice, 7,* 373–385. doi:10.1093/clipsy.7.4.373

Santangelo, P., Reinhard, I., Mussgay, L., Steil, R., Sawitzki, G., Klein, C., ... Ebner-Priemer, U. W. (2014). Specificity of affective instability in patients with borderline personality disorder compared to posttraumatic stress disorder, bulimia nervosa, and healthy controls. *Journal of Abnormal Psychology, 123,* 258–272. doi:10.1037/a0035619

Schienle, A., Haas-Krammer, A., Schöggl, H., Kapfhammer, H.-P., & Ille, R. (2013). Altered state and trait disgust in borderline personality disorder. *Journal of Nervous and Mental Disease, 201,* 105–108. doi:10.1097/NMD.0b013e31827f64da

Silk, K. R. (2010). The quality of depression in borderline personality disorder and the diagnostic process. *Journal of Personality Disorders, 24,* 25–37. doi:10.1521/pedi.2010.24.1.25

Taskforce OPD. (2008). *Operationalized Psychodynamic Diagnostics OPD-2: Manual of diagnosis and treatment planning.* Cambridge, MA: Hogrefe.

Thayer, R. E. (1989). *The biopsychology of mood and arousal.* New York, NY: Oxford University Press.

Tingley, D., Yamamoto, T., Hirose, K., Keele, L., & Imai, K. (2014). Mediation: R package for causal mediation analysis. *Journal of Statistical Software, 59*(5), 1–39. Retrieved from http://hdl.handle.net/1721.1/91154

Trull, T. J., & Durrett, C. A. (2005). Categorical and dimensional models of personality disorder. *Annual Review of Clinical Psychology, 1*(1), 355–380. doi:10.1146/annurev.clinpsy.1.102803.144009

Tyrer, P., Crawford, M., Mulder, R., Blashfield, R., Farnam, A., Fossati, A., . . . Reed, G. M. (2011). The rationale for the reclassification of personality disorder in the 11th revision of the International Classification of Diseases (ICD‐11). *Personality and Mental Health. 5*, 246–259. doi:10.1002/pmh.190

Unger, T., Hoffmann, S., Köhler, S., Mackert, A., & Fydrich, T. (2013). Personality disorders and outcome of inpatient treatment for depression: A 1-year prospective follow-up study. *Journal of Personality Disorders, 27*, 636–651. doi:10.1521/pedi_2012_26_052

Waugh, M. H., Hopwood, C. J., Krueger, R. F., Morey, L. C., Pincus, A. L., & Wright, A. G. C. (2017). Psychological assessment with the *DSM-5* alternative model for personality disorders: Tradition and innovation. *Professional Psychology Research and Practice, 48*, 79–89. doi:10.1037/pro0000071

Westen, D., Moses, M. J., Silk, K. R., Lohr, N. E., Cohen, R., & Segal, H. (1992). Quality of depressive experience in borderline personality disorder and major depression: When depression is not just depression. *Journal of Personality Disorders, 6*, 382–393. doi:10.1521/pedi.1992.6.4.382

Zanarini, M. C., & Frankenburg, F. R. (2007). The essential nature of borderline psychopathology. *Journal of Personality Disorders, 21*, 518–535. doi:10.1521/pedi.2007.21.5.518

Zimmermann, J., Benecke, C., Bender, D. S., Skodol, A. E., Schauenburg, H., Cierpka, M., & Leising, D. (2014). Assessing *DSM-5* level of personality functioning from videotaped clinical interviews: A pilot study with untrained and clinically inexperienced students. *Journal of Personality Assessment, 96*, 397–409. doi:10.1080/00223891.2013.852563

Zimmermann, J., Böhnke, J. R., Eschstruth, R., Mathews, A., Wenzel, K., & Leising, D. (2015). The latent structure of personality functioning: Investigating Criterion A from the alternative model for personality disorders in *DSM-5*. Journal of Abnormal Psychology, 124, 532–548. doi:10.1037/abn0000059

Zimmermann, J., Dahlbender, R. W., Herbold, W., Krasnow, K., Turrión, C. M., Zika, M., & Spitzer, C. (2015). The OPD Structure Questionnaire captures the general features of personality disorder. *Psychotherapie, Psychosomatik, medizinische Psychologie, 65*, 81–83. doi:10.1016/0010-440X(92)90010-N

Zimmermann, J., Ehrenthal, J. C., Cierpka, M., Schauenburg, H., Doering, S., & Benecke, C. (2012). Assessing the level of structural integration using Operationalized Psychodynamic Diagnosis (OPD): Implications for *DSM-5*. *Journal of Personality Assessment, 94*, 522–532. doi:10.1080/00223891.2012.700664

Exploring the Effectiveness of Dialectical Behavior Therapy versus Systems Training for Emotional Predictability and Problem Solving in a Sample of Patients with Borderline Personality Disorder

Verónica Guillén Botella, PhD, Azucena García-Palacios, PhD, Sara Bolo Miñana, MClinPsych, Rosa Baños, PhD, Cristina Botella, PhD, and José Heliodoro Marco, PhD

> Dialectical behavior therapy (DBT) and systems training for emotional predictability and problem solving (STEPPS) are two treatment protocols for people with borderline personality disorder (BPD) that have received important empirical support. However, their possible differential effectiveness has not yet been studied. The objective of this study is to explore the effectiveness of these two treatment programs. A nonrandomized clinical trial was carried out in which both treatments were applied for six months. The sample consisted of 72 patients diagnosed with BPD. The results indicate that both groups experienced a statistically significant reduction in BPD symptom, emotional regulation, impulsiveness, dissociative experiences, suicidal risk, depression, or anger. However, the DBT condition obtained statistically significant differences in BPD behavioral symptoms and fear of suicide. DBT and STEPPS treatment are effective treatments for participants with BPD, and DBT was more effective for the behavioral symptoms of BPD.
>
> *Keywords:* personality disorder, borderline personality disorder, psychological treatment, dialectical behavior therapy, systems training for emotional predictability and problem solving

Borderline personality disorder (BPD) is the personality disorder for which the most progress has been made in the past 30 years. Currently, its treatment has important empirical support from different orientations. According to the American Psychiatric Association (APA), at present, dialectical behavioral

---

From Universidad de Valencia, Valencia, Spain (V. G. B., S. B. M., R. B., J. H. M.); Universitat Jaume I de Castellón, Castellón, Spain (A. G.-P., C. B.); and Ciber Fisiopatologia Obesidad y Nutricion (CB06/03 Instituto Salud Carlos III), Madrid, Spain (V. G. B., A. G.-P., R. B., C. B.).

The authors would like to acknowledge the Personality Disorders Unit, Previ, Valencia, Spain.

Address correspondence to Verónica Guillén Botella, Department of Personality, Evaluation and Psychological Treatments, University of Valencia, Av. Blasco Ibañez 21, Spain, 46010. E-mail: veronica.guillen@uv.es

---

Originally published in the *Journal of Personality Disorders*, Volume 35, Supplement A. ©2021 The Guilford Press.

therapy (DBT) is the treatment of choice for BPD, with more than 40 randomized control trials (APA, 2013). DBT was initially developed to address emotion dysregulation and suicidal and parasuicidal behaviors in people with BPD (Linehan, 2014). The original DBT program consists of four group skills-training modules (mindfulness, interpersonal effectiveness, emotion regulation, and distress tolerance modules), individual therapy, telephone crisis coaching, and a therapist consultation team (Linehan, 2014). Recent meta-analyses have established the efficacy of DBT for a variety of mental health problems, including BPD (Cristea et al., 2017), and DBT has been adapted for use in other psychiatric conditions, such as eating disorders, including anorexia nervosa, bulimia nervosa (Safer, Telch, & Agras, 2001), or binge-eating disorders (Linardon, Fairburn, Fitzsimmons-Craft, Wilfley, & Brennan, 2017; Linardon, Gleeson, Yap, Murphy, & Brennan, 2019), and suicidal behaviors (DeCou, Comtois, & Landes, 2019), as well as other psychiatric conditions such as mood disorders (Burckhardt et al., 2018), posttraumatic stress disorder (Bohus et al., 2013), or comorbid disorders (Harned, Korslund, & Linehan, 2014). However, DBT interventions require high therapist specialization, which is sometimes not possible due to its high costs in terms of time and money. Finally, the main limitation is usually the difficulty of implementing standard DBT in mental health services (Blum, Pfohl, John, Monahan, & Blank, 2002).

Another cognitive-behavioral intervention that has received empirical support is systems training for emotional predictability and problem solving (STEPPS), developed by Nancy Blum (Blum et al., 2002). STEPPS is a manual-based 20-week group therapy for individuals with BPD that includes psychoeducation about BPD, cognitive-behavioral techniques, and behavior management training, such as goal setting, lifestyle behaviors, and interpersonal skills. STEPPS has demonstrated promising empirical support across several settings. In general, it is recommended for reducing BPD symptom severity, depressive symptoms, and general psychiatric symptoms. Two studies from different research sites (Blum et al., 2002; Harvey, Black, & Blum, 2010) show that STEPPS reduces self-reported and clinician-rated BPD symptom severity. One RCT has also compared STEPPS plus treatment-as-usual (TAU) to TAU alone, and the results showed that STEPPS achieves greater improvements in clinician-rated BPD symptom severity, compared to TAU, with a large effect size difference maintained at follow-up (Blum et al., 2008). A Dutch version of STEPPS plus a STEPPS-focused individual psychotherapy compared to TAU also resulted in greater improvements in BPD symptoms, with a medium effect size difference that was maintained at follow-up (Bos, van Wel, Appelo, & Verbraak, 2010). STEPPS has also been studied in forensic groups, such as prisoners with BPD, and findings showed that STEPPS resulted in reductions in BPD severity with a large effect size from baseline to the end of treatment (Black, Blum, McCormick, & Allen, 2013). STEPPS has been tested in the treatment of bipolar disorder and comorbid personality features (Reimann et al., 2014).

STEPPS is also a long treatment. The patients usually perform the group therapy sequence once or twice, but it does not require a high level of specialization (Blum et al., 2002). One of the goals when developing STEPPS was to create a program that would require little additional training for mental health professionals, given the limited time they have. STEPPS includes general psychotherapy principles and techniques common to most psychotherapy educational programs, and so therapists with widely varying educational and professional backgrounds can use it. Usually, a therapist who is an expert in cognitive-behavioral therapy and has experience in BPD can take a 1-to-2-day workshop on site and be prepared to run groups. In addition, the manualized psychoeducational STEPPS procedure allows this program to be implemented fairly easily in community health care settings (Fitzpatrick, Wagner, & Monson, 2019).

Despite the good data on DBT and STEPPS, these programs also have some limitations. Although numerous RCTs using DBT have been published, in many studies this treatment program is compared with a waiting list condition (Safer et al., 2001) or with TAU (Blum et al., 2008; Linehan, Armstrong, Suarez, Allmon, & Heard, 1991; Priebe et al., 2012) or a delayed-treatment control (Hill, Craighead, & Safer, 2011). Few studies have compared the differential efficacy of the application of DBT with other active treatment programs, such as DBT versus mentalization-based treatment (MBT) (Barnicot & Crawford, 2019). Thus, it is necessary to compare DBT versus other active treatment programs, in order to evaluate which is more effective in resolving specific problems. Comparing different programs can also help to advance in personalizing treatments by providing more information about the patients for whom each program works better. Finally, it is also important to explore the clinical contexts where different programs can be implemented.

The main objective of this study is to assess, in an open clinical trial, the effectiveness of a treatment protocol based on DBT, compared to a treatment protocol based on STEPPS, in a sample of patients diagnosed with BPD. Considering the data in the literature, the initial hypothesis is that both programs will be effective and can be implemented in a personality disorder unit, although DBT will achieve better results than the protocol based on STEPPS.

METHOD

Participants

The sample was composed of 72 patients from three specialized Personality Disorder Units in Spain. The inclusion criteria were patients who (a) met the criteria in the fifth edition of the *Diagnostic and Statistical Manual of Mental Disorders* (*DSM-5*; APA, 2013) for BPD and (b) accepted the treatment. The exclusion criteria were (a) moderate or severe intellectual disability and (b) a diagnosis of schizophrenia or bipolar disorder. Written informed consent was obtained during the inclusion interview. All participants were Caucasian, and they received no compensation. Ethical approval for this study was granted by the Previ Foundation Ethics Committee. Participants were consecutively recruited. In the sample, 94.4% were women, $n = 68$, and 5.6% men, $n = 4$. The participants' ages ranged from 14 to 60 years, with a mean of 32.12 ($SD = 8.83$). Table 1 and Table 2 show the participants' sociodemographic and clinical characteristics.

TABLE 1. Sociodemographic Characteristics of the Participants in the Two Treatment Conditions

	DBT		STEPPS		Total	
	n = 45	%	n = 27	%	N = 72	%
Sex						
Male	3	6.7	0	0	3	5.2
Female	42	93.3	27	100.0	69	94.8
Education level						
Elementary education	13	29.0	13	48.1	26	37.9
Middle education	22	48.4	11	40.7	33	44.8
Higher education	10	22.6	3	11.1	13	17.3
Marital status						
Single	35	77.4	18	66.7	53	72.8
Married	4	9.7	5	18.5	9	12.9
Divorced	6	12.9	4	14.8	10	14.3
Age						
14–20 years	6	12.9	2	7.4	8	10.3
21–30 years	19	41.9	6	22.2	25	32.8
31–40 years	13	29.0	13	48.1	26	37.9
41–50 years	7	16.1	6	22.2	13	19.0

Note: DBT = dialectical behavior therapy; STEPPS = Systems Training for Emotional Predictability and Problem Solving; n = number of participants.

Measures

We selected the primary and secondary outcomes based on previous RCT with BPD (e.g., McMain, Guimond, Barnhart, Habinski, & Streiner, 2017). The primary outcomes were changes in typical emotional BPD symptoms and changes in typical behavioral BPD symptoms, assessed with the Borderline Symptom List 23 (BSL-23) (Bohus et al., 2008). The BSL-23 is a reliable and valid self-report instrument for assessing BPD severity (Soler et al., 2013). The Spanish version of the BSL-23 (Soler et al., 2013) is composed of 23 items measured on a Likert scale (five response levels) related to different BPD symptoms. It also includes a supplementary 11-item Likert scale (five response levels) to assess the frequency of behaviors characteristic of BPD in the past week: nonsuicidal self-injuries, suicide threat, suicide attempt, binge eating,

TABLE 2. Clinical Characteristics of the Participants in the Two Treatment Conditions

	DBT	STEPPS	Total
Hospitalizations lifetime	3.95 (4.29)	2.17 (4.01)	3.57 (4.23)
Hospitalizations last 6 months	0.27 (0.63)	0.17 (0.41)	0.25 (0.58)
Suicide attempts lifetime	2.32 (2.29)	0.83 (1.17)	2 (2.17)
Suicide attempts last 6 months	0.09 (0.29)	0.17 (0.41)	0.11 (0.31)
Global Assessment Functioning	55.56 (8.97)	62.92 (12.34)	59.24 (11.30)
Severity of participants index	7.58 (1.71)	5.80 (1.07)	6.62 (1.65)

Note: All values are M (SD). DBT = dialectical behavior therapy; STEPPS = Systems Training for Emotional Predictability and Problem Solving.

purging, high-risk behaviors, getting drunk, drug use, mediation overdose, aggressive behavior, and sexual impulsivity. The Spanish version of the BSL-23 replicates the one-factor structure of the original version (Soler et al., 2013). The scale has excellent internal consistency (Cronbach's alpha = .949), as well as good test-retest stability, which was checked in a subsample after one week ($n = 74$; $r = .734$; $p < .01$) (George & Mallery, 2003).

The secondary outcomes were changes in the general BPD psychopathology and changes in coping skills. Table 3 shows the secondary outcomes.

Moreover, to assess the severity of the participants, we used two different measures. First, the global assessment of functioning (GAF) from the fourth edition of the *DSM* (*DSM-IV*; APA, 2000), which is the standard method for representing a clinician's judgment of a patient's current psychological, social, and occupational functioning. The GAF is composed of a scale from 1 to 100, with ratings from 1 to 10 indicating severe impairment, and ratings from 91 to 100 indicating superior functioning. The GAF is accepted as a reliable and valid measure (Jones, Thornicroft, Coffey, & Dunn, 1995). Second, the severity of participants index, a single item that assesses the opinion of the therapist about the severity of the participant's psychopathology (range 0–10); 0 is absence of severity, and 10 is high severity.

Study Design

This study is a two-group, multiple site, nonrandomized clinical trial performed in a naturalistic setting. Two experimental conditions were used.

TABLE 3. Secondary Measures

Instrument	Spanish version	Items	Constructs measured	Reliability
Beck Depression Inventory-II (BDI-II; Beck, Steer, & Brown, 1996)	Sanz, Perdigón, & Vazquez (2003)	21	Depression	Good ($\alpha = 0.87$)
Barratt Impulsivity Scale (BIS-11; Patton, Stanford, & Barratt, 1995)	Oquendo et al. (2001)	30	Impulsivity	Good ($\alpha = 0.83$)
Dissociative Experiences Scale-II (DES-II; Carlson & Putnam, 1993)	Icarán, Colom, & Orengo-García (1996)	28	Dissociation	Excellent ($\alpha = 0.95$)
Overall Anxiety Severity and Impairment Scale (OASIS; Norman, Cissell, Means-Christensen, & Stein, 2006)	González-Robles et al. (2018)	5	Anxiety	Good ($\alpha = 0.80$)
Suicide Risk Scale (SRS; Plutchik, Van Praag, Cone, & Picard, 1989)	Rubio et al. (1998)	15	Risk of suicide	Excellent ($\alpha = 0.92$)
State-Trait Anger Expression Inventory—II (STAXI-II; Spielberger, 1999)	Miguel-Tobal, Casado, Cano-Vindel, & Spielberger (2001)	49	Anger	Range ($\alpha = 0.66$ to 0.88)
Quality of Life Index (QoL; Mezzich et al., 2000)	Mezzich et al. (2000)	10	Quality of life	Acceptable ($\alpha = 0.79$)
Difficulties in Emotional Regulation Scale (DERS; Gratz & Roemer, 2004)	Hervás & Jodar (2008)	28	Difficulties in emotional regulation	Excellent ($\alpha = 0.91$)
Resilience Scale-15 (RS-15; Wilks, 2008)	Wilks (2008)	15	Resilience	Excellent ($\alpha = 0.91$)
Reasons for Living (RFL; Linehan, Goodstein, Nielsen, & Chiles, 1983)	Oquendo et al. (2000)	48	Reasons for living	Good (range $\alpha = 0.72$ to 0.89)

Intervention Protocol Based on DBT for Patients With BPD. In this condition, the manualized DBT treatment for BPD was applied (Linehan, 1993a, 1993b). Regarding the structure of the therapy, the DBT condition was composed of skills training (group format), individual psychotherapy, telephone consultations, consultations with other professionals, auxiliary treatments, and 2-hour weekly clinician meetings for supervision. The treatment was applied in 24 sessions of group therapy, consisting of a weekly session lasting 2 hours, and individual therapy in a weekly 1-hour session. With a total of 48 hours of group therapy and 24 hours of individual therapy, the two modalities (individual and group) added up to a total of 72 hours of treatment.

Intervention Protocol Based on STEPPS. In this condition, the STEPPS program for BPD was applied (Blum et al., 2002). It was composed of group therapy, the reinforcement team, telephone consultations with relatives, consultations with other professionals, and weekly clinician meetings. The program was carried out in 20-week group therapy, consisting of a weekly session lasting 2 hours; and it included a 1-hour session of individual psychotherapy during the 20 weeks. Moreover, STEPPS incorporates one session (2 hours) for the reinforcement team, which involves informing family and friends about BPD, STEPPS skills content, and strategies to encourage the individual with BPD to use his or her newly acquired skills. With a total of 40 hours of group therapy and 20 hours of individual therapy, the two modalities (individual and group therapy) added up to a total of 60 hours of treatment.

In both cases, the standard therapy for each orientation was used. However, the STEPPS program was complemented with individual therapy in order to balance the two conditions.

Procedure

The treatments were carried out in the Personality Disorder Unit. This unit offers individualized, integral, and multidisciplinary treatment (psychological, psychiatric, socio-occupational, etc.) for people who suffer from BPD and their families. Evaluation and treatment are approached from a biopsychosocial perspective. An exhaustive psychological evaluation is performed to evaluate the diagnosis and clinical severity and establish the therapeutic plan. Patients diagnosed with BPD who were already undergoing treatment at the clinical center were offered the opportunity to participate in the study. Once the study had been explained to them, they completed and signed the informed consent, and several clinical psychologists, experts in BPD, carried out the assessment of the patients to verify that they met the inclusion and exclusion criteria. Two psychological evaluation sessions were necessary to carry out the assessment protocol. In the first session, it was confirmed that the participants met the inclusion criteria, the objective of the study was explained, and the participants signed the consent form. The researchers established the participants' diagnosis using the diagnostic criteria of the *DSM-5* (APA, 2013). In the second session, the assessment protocol was filled out. The patients completed this protocol two times: pre- and posttreatment. Moreover, a feedback interview with the patient or his or her family (for adolescents below the age of 18) was conducted to inform patients or their relatives. In this interview, the patients or the family members were given information about the diagnosis, prognosis, and most appropriate intervention in their case. Regarding the decision about the type of intervention, the clinical team proposed the most appropriate type of intervention for each patient based on the diagnosis and current state of the disorder. The treatment in the unit consisted of 1 hour of individual therapy per week and group therapy, such as DBT skills training or a STEPPS group.

The usual procedure at the clinical center is the following. For the more severe BPD cases (severe emotion dysregulation and severe suicidal and parasuicidal behaviors, eating disorder comorbidities, mood disorders, substance abuse, comorbidities, etc.) or long-term patients, the DBT program is recommended. In cases with less BPD symptomatology, treatments with shorter duration, or younger patients, the STEPPS therapy group is recommended to reduce BPD symptoms, depressive symptoms, and general psychiatric symptoms. So far, the literature does not provide indication for assigning different patients to one treatment program or another. In the three clinical centers where the study was carried out, the procedure was similar. Patients were consecutively assigned to an experimental condition until the group was complete (e.g., DBT), and then they were assigned consecutively to the other experimental condition (e.g., STEPPS). Each group was directed by two therapists (a therapist and cotherapist), with a total of 12 therapists in the three facilities. All the therapists were expert psychologists in the treatment of personality disorders and each had more than 10 years of experience. All of them had at least a master's degree in clinical psychology. The therapists had received training in DBT and had been applying it for at least 10 years. Regarding STEPPS, the therapists had received the 2-day training and had been applying it for 6 years. To confirm the integrity of the treatments without disturbing the functioning of the clinical center, supervision sessions were carried out, and both treatment protocols were manualized. It should be noted that, because the therapists had received previous training in DBT and STEPPS, these group therapies have been routinely applied in the clinical centers. Regarding the assignment of the therapists in general in the center, the groups rotate among the different therapists. For this study, the therapists who were running DBT groups conducted the DBT groups, and those who were running STEPPS groups conducted the STEPPS groups.

Data Analysis

In order to analyze whether there were differences between the experimental conditions before the application of the treatment, Student's t tests were performed for the continuous variables, as well as Mann-Whitney U test for the categorical variables. To compare the effectiveness of the two treatment conditions, we performed a multivariate analysis of variance for repeated measures (MANOVA) for the variables with subscales, and ANOVA for the single variables, taking the pretreatment and posttreatment moments as within-subject factor and the treatment condition (DBT versus STEPPS) as between-subject factor. We performed the MANOVA and ANOVA with, age, severity, and educational level as covariates. All analyses were performed with the SPSS version 24.

RESULTS

Participant Flow

As Figure 1 shows, 77 participants were evaluated, and 5 were excluded because they did not meet all the inclusion criteria. Finally, 72 participants were assigned to the two experimental conditions. In the DBT condition, there were 14 (31.1%) dropouts, and in the STEPPS condition, there were 9 (33.3%) dropouts. A dropout was defined as a patient who does not complete at least 80% of the therapy sessions or does not perform the posttreatment assessment.

Differences Between Conditions Before And After Treatment

As Table 1 shows, there were no differences in age, $t(56) = -1.49$; $p = .46$; gender, Mann-Whitney $U = 378$, $p = .10$; educational level, Mann-Whitney $U = 322.5$, $p = .11$; or marital status, Mann-Whitney $U = 377.5$, $p = .41$. Moreover, Table 2 reveals that there were no differences in lifetime hospitalizations,

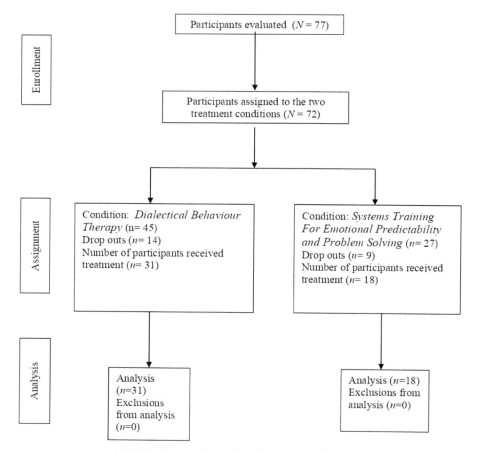

FIGURE 1. Sample Evolution Throughout Treatment.

$t(28) = .78$, $p = .91$; hospitalizations in the past 6 months, $t(28) = .32$, $p = .75$; lifetime suicide attempts, $t(28) = 1.68$, $p = .10$; or suicide attempts in the past 6 months, $t(28) = -.59$, $p = .56$. However, the participants in the DBT condition had lower GAF, $t(48) = 2.41$, $p < .02$, and higher severity, $t(48) = 4.05$, $p < .001$, than the participants in the STEPPS condition. Therefore, the clinicians rated the DBT participants as more severe than the STEPPS participants.

Table 4 presents the mean and standard deviations for all the measures before and after the psychotherapy. Moreover, the table shows the differences

TABLE 4. Participants' Pretreatment and Posttreatment Scores, and Differences Between the Two Treatment Conditions at Pretreatment

	DBT condition		STEPPS condition		Differences between conditions before treatment	
	Pretreatment M (SD)	Posttreatment M (SD)	Pretreatment M (SD)	Posttreatment M (SD)	t	p
Primary outcomes						
Borderline symptoms (BSL)	35.78 (22.73)	23.56 (29.25)	38.59 (20.24)	29.29 (23.76)	−.13	.89
Behavioral subscale (BSL)	5.2 (5.88)	2.60 (4.22)	3.81 (2.93)	4.31 (3.75)	.85	.40
Secondary outcomes						
Depression (BDI)	36.32 (15.08)	28.03 (17.45)	28.94 (11.87)	21.33 (12.96)	1.71	.09
Cognitive impulsiveness (BIS)	12.93 (2.73)	11.57 (3.82)	14.53 (3.12)	13.37 (3.80)	−1.55	.13
Motor impulsiveness (BIS)	14.57 (4.47)	12.29 (5.54)	16.95 (3.73)	14.84 (5.85)	−1.46	.15
Nonplanned impulsiveness (BIS)	14.64 (4.88)	13.79 (5.01)	17.32 (5.89)	16.21 (6.21)	−1.09	.82
Attention (DERS)	13.10 (4.04)	8.80 (3.52)	12.53 (4.03)	11.47 (3.45)	0.68	.49
Clarity (DERS)	13.10 (4.82)	8.20 (4.26)	12.47 (3.79)	10.74 (4.86)	0.80	.42
Acceptance (DERS)	21.20 (7.66)	15.80 (9.27)	25.68 (8.37)	20.16 (10.48)	−1.36	.18
Functioning (DERS)	14.60 (4.60)	12.60 (5.97)	15.89 (3.74)	13.42 (4.41)	6.86	.49
Regulation (DERS)	28.90 (7.96)	20.00 (11.80)	30.53 (8.53)	23.21 (9.07)	−2.24	.81
Dissociation (DES-II)	26.02 (14.13)	20.81 (17.01)	24.19 (14.76)	17.99 (13.94)	1.04	.30
Quality of life (QoL)	4.37 (1.71)	6.31 (2.31)	4.26 (1.74)	5.15 (1.49)	0.22	.82
Anxiety (OASIS)	10.60 (5.58)	8.40 (6.11)	10.05 (5.28)	9.11 (5.01)	0.11	.91
Suicidal risk (SRS)	9.20 (3.77)	7.00 (4.83)	10.17 (2.57)	8.56 (3.15)	−0.68	.51
Resilience (RS-15)	54.20 (19.38)	70.70 (24.50)	51.79 (17.60)	58.16 (17.66)	0.09	.92
Anger state (STAXI)	29.38 (12.00)	25.76 (12.93)	29.39 (12.17)	23.67 (10.36)	0.85	.39
Anger trait (STAXI)	27.41 (6.37)	22.72 (8.26)	31.61 (6.71)	25.78 (7.29)	−1.79	.08
Anger expression (STAXI)	45.24 (10.87)	32.31 (13.63)	41.94 (10.82)	35.28 (12.17)	−0.04	.97
Survival coping beliefs (RFL)	3.72 (.99)	3.96 (1.51)	3.49 (1.13)	3.77 (1.26)	0.69	.49
Responsibility to family (RFL)	4.16 (.65)	4.34 (1.15)	4.51 (1.37)	4.48 (1.44)	−0.59	.55
Child-related concerns (RFL)	3.63 (2.12)	2.81 (2.10)	3.15 (2.21)	3.00 (2.36)	−0.20	.98
Fear of suicide (RFL)	2.92 (1.07)	2.59 (1.28)	2.65 (1.20)	3.09 (1.29)	0.47	.63
Fear of social disapproval (RFL)	3.10 (1.63)	3.33 (2.14)	2.94 (1.77)	2.48 (1.12)	0.17	.41
Moral objections (RFL)	2.23 (1.57)	1.70 (.99)	1.69 (1.11)	1.72 (1.06)	0.86	.39

Note: BDI = Beck Depression Inventory-II; BIS = Barratt Impulsiveness Scale; BSL-23 = Borderline Symptom List-23; DERS = Difficulties in Emotion Regulation Scale; DES-II = Dissociative Experiences Scale-II; QoL= Quality of Life; OASIS = Overall Anxiety Severity and Impairment Scale; SRS = Suicide Risk Scale; RS-15 = Resilience Scale; STAXI = State-Trait Anger Expression Inventor-II; RFL = Reasons for Living; DBT = dialectical behavior therapy; STEPPS = Systems Training for Emotional Predictability and Problem Solving.

in the measures between the two treatment conditions at pretreatment. For the primary outcomes, there were no statistically significant differences in borderline symptoms, and for the secondary outcomes, there were no statistically significant differences in general BPD psychopathology and coping skills between the two treatment conditions before starting the treatment.

Regarding comorbidities with other mental disorders, in the sample of patients in the DBT condition, 61.29%, $n = 19$, met feeding and eating disorder criteria; 16.12%, $n = 5$, met substance use disorder criteria; 6.45%, $n = 2$, met posttraumatic stress disorder criteria; 3.22%, $n = 1$, met major depressive disorder criteria; and 12.92%, $n = 4$, had no comorbidities. Of the participants in the STEPPS condition, 14.81%, $n = 4$, met the criteria for feeding and eating disorders; 7.40%, $n = 2$, for major depressive disorder; 3.70%, $n = 1$, for attention-deficit hyperactivity disorder; and 74.09%, $n = 20$, had no comorbidity with another mental disorder. Thus, the DBT participants had more comorbidity than the STEPPS participants.

Pretreatment versus Posttreatment Differences

Primary Outcomes. As Table 5 reveals, the DBT condition showed more improvement in borderline symptomatology than the STEPPS condition, $F(1,45) = 7.39$, $p = .03$, $\mu^2 = .30$. Specifically, on the behavioral subscale of borderline symptoms (BSL-23), both conditions improved after treatment, $F(1, 45) = 4.98$, $p = 03$, $\mu^2 = .20$, but the DBT condition showed more improvement than the STEPPS condition (BSL-23, $F(1, 45) = 8.42$, $p = .01$, $\mu^2 = .30$.

Secondary Outcomes. Table 5 shows that both treatment conditions (DBT and STEPPS) demonstrated a statistically significant improvement from pretreatment to posttreatment on the fear of suicide subscale (RFL), $F(1, 45) = 4.74$, $p = .04$, $\mu^2 = .19$, but the DBT condition showed more improvement than the STEPPS condition, $F(1, 45) = 8.62$, $p = .01$, $\mu^2 = .30$.

Moreover, both treatment conditions (DBT and STEPPS) showed a statistically significant improvement from pretreatment to posttreatment in the psychopathology of BPD related to: emotional deregulation, $F(1, 48) = 3.75$, $p = .05$, $\mu^2 = .48$, specifically on the emotional regulation subscale (DERS), $F(1, 48) = 7.48$, $p = .01$, $\mu^2 = .24$; dissociation (DES-II), $F(1, 48) = 5.09$, $p = .03$, $\mu^2 = .03$; anxiety (OASIS), $F(1, 48) = 7.35$, $p = .01$, $\mu^2 = .23$; suicidal risk (SRS), $F(1, 48) = 4.63$, $p = .04$, $\mu^2 = .17$; and anger trait (STAXI), $F(1, 45) = 4.45$, $p = .04$, $\mu^2 = .10$. However, on these variables, there were no statistically significant differences between the two treatment conditions at the end of treatment.

As Table 5 shows, there were no statistically significant differences between the two treatment conditions on the rest of the measures at the end of treatment.

TABLE 5. Differences Between the Two Treatment Conditions Before and After the Treatment

	Multivariate analysis						Univariate analysis						Posttreatment differences between groups
	Pre-post			DBT vs. STEPPS			Pre-post			DBT vs. STEPPS			
	F	p	η^2	F	p	η^2	F	p	η^2	F	p	η^2	
Primary outcomes													
Borderline symptoms	2.63	.09	.22	7.39*	.03	.30							DBT < STEPPS
Borderline symptoms (BSL)							0.70	.41	.03	0.15	.70	.01	
Behavioral subscale (BSL)							4.98*	.03	.20	8.42*	.01	.30	DBT < STEPPS
Secondary outcomes													
Depression (BDI)							0.27	.60	.01	0.03	.87	.01	
Impulsiveness	0.47	.70	.05	0.36	.78	.04							
Cognitive impulsiveness (BIS)							0.45	.50	.02	0.01	.99	.01	
Motor impulsiveness (BIS)							0.51	.47	.02	0.01	.78	.01	
Nonplanned impulsiveness (BIS)							0.96	.33	.03	0.01	.24	.01	
Emotional deregulation	3.75*	.01	.48	1.10	.38	.22							
Attention (DERS)							3.27	.08	.12	0.77	.38	.03	
Clarity (DERS)							0.11	.74	.01	2.17	.15	.09	
Acceptance (DERS)							2.61	.11	.09	0.05	.81	.01	
Functioning (DERS)							3.06	.09	.11	1.01	.32	.04	
Regulation (DERS)							7.48*	.01	.24	0.21	.65	.01	
Dissociation (DES - II)							5.09*	.03	14	0.31	.86	.01	
Quality of life (QoL)							0.41	.52	.02	1.22	.28	.05	
Anxiety (OASIS)							7.35*	.01	.23	2.27	.14	.08	
Suicidal Risk Scale (SRS)							4.63*	.04	.17	0.05	.08	.01	
Resilience (RS-15)							2.70	.11	.10	0.94	.76	.01	
Anger deregulation	1.46	.24	.10	0.36	.78	.03							
Anger state (STAXI)							0.24	.62	.10	0.76	.38	.02	
Anger trait (STAXI)							4.45*	.04	.10	0.68	.41	.02	
Anger expression (STAXI)							18.6		.29	0.29	.59	.01	
Reasons for Living	0.98	.47	.28	2.73	.05	.52							
Survival coping beliefs (RFL)							2.4	.13	.11	0.18	.67	.01	
Responsibility to family (RFL)							1.02	.32	.05	0.01	.92	.01	
Child-related concerns (RFL)							0.47	.49	.02	0.51	.48	.02	
Fear of suicide (RFL)							4.74*	.04	.19	8.62*	.01	.30	DBT < STEPPS
Fear of social disapproval (RFL)							0.15	.70	.01	0.97	.33	.04	
Moral objections (RFL)							3.39	.08	.14	3.86	.06	.16	

Note: BDI = Beck Depression Inventory-II; BIS = Barratt Impulsiveness Scale; BSL-23 = Borderline Symptom List-23; DERS = Difficulties in Emotion Regulation Scale; DES-II = Dissociative Experiences Scale-II; QoL= Quality of Life; OASIS = Overall Anxiety Severity and Impairment Scale; SRS = Suicide Risk Scale; RS-15 = Resilience Scale; STAXI = State-Trait Anger Expression Inventory-II; RFL = Reasons for Living; DBT = dialectical behavior therapy; STEPPS = Systems Training for Emotional Predictability and Problem Solving; DBT < STEPPS = at posttreatment, the DBT condition showed lower scores than the STEPPS condition. *p < .05.

DISCUSSION

The objective of this study was to explore the effectiveness, in an open clinical trial, of a treatment protocol based on DBT, compared to a treatment protocol based on STEPPS, for 72 patients with BPD. In both cases, we used the standard therapy for each orientation. In the DBT condition, we used 24 sessions of skills training, individual psychotherapy, telephone consultations with relatives, consultations with other professionals, auxiliary treatments, and 2-hour weekly clinician meetings. In the STEPPS condition, we used 20 sessions of group therapy, one session with the reinforcement team, telephone consultations with relatives, consultations with other professionals, and weekly clinician meetings. We added individual psychotherapy in order to balance the amount of therapy received in the two conditions. In both conditions, group therapy sessions were carried out on a weekly basis and lasted 2 hours. The participants in the DBT condition received a total of 72 hours (individual and group therapy) of treatment, and participants in the STEPPS condition received 60 hours. Considering the clinical severity of these patients and the long duration these treatments usually have, we do not think this difference in treatment hours is an important issue.

There were no statistically significant differences between the two treatment conditions before the treatment in any of the variables considered in the evaluation, except in the number of mental disorder comorbidities, and the severity rated by the clinicians (GAF). The DBT group had more patients with eating disorders, substance abuse, mood disorders, and posttraumatic stress disorder, and their GAF ratings were lower. Therefore, the sample of patients in the DBT group was more severe.

The results indicate that both conditions showed a statistically significant improvement from pretreatment to posttreatment (DBT and STEPPS) on important measures such as BPD symptom severity, emotional regulation, and dissociative experiences. Both groups had a statistically significant reduction in suicidal risk, anxiety, or anger, along the same lines as other studies in the literature (Andreasson et al., 2016; Blum et al., 2002, 2008; Bos et al., 2012; Harned et al., 2014).

However, the DBT condition obtained statistically significant differences in key variables such as BPD behavioral symptoms (e.g., suicide attempts, nonsuicidal self-injuries, etc.) and fear of suicide, coinciding with other studies (Blum et al., 2008; Bos et al., 2010; McMain et al., 2009; Neacsiu, Lungu, Harned, Rizvi, & Linehan, 2014; Pasieczny & Connor, 2011). Moreover, there is a trend in favor of the DBT program on variables such as emotional regulation, resilience, and quality of life that did not reach statistical significance, perhaps due to the small sample size or because the DBT group was worse than the STEPPS group before starting treatment, in terms of comorbidity and severity. In this regard, it is important to note that, in both conditions, there were no differences in biographical variables (age, gender, educational level, or marital status) before beginning the treatment. Nevertheless, the participants in the DBT condition had lower GAF and higher severity than the participants in the STEPPS condition, and the clinicians rated the DBT participants as more severe than the STEPPS participants. On the other hand, in both cases, the standard therapy for each orientation was used, and the STEPPS program was complemented with individual therapy in order to balance the two conditions. The difference in total hours of the treatments does not seem significant considering that the participants in this study had personality disorders.

In this study, the dropout rates were quite similar in the DBT group (31.1%) and STEPPS group (33.3%), and there were no statistically significant differences between them, unlike in other studies where different dropout rates were found (Dixon & Linardon, 2019). Moreover, dropout rates were quite similar to those presented in the literature. For example, Landes, Chalker, and Comtois (2016) found that the dropout rate in outpatient DBT in the community can be as high as 24% to 58%.

These results are in line with those found by Barnicot and Crawford (2019), where they compared DBT versus MBT in a nonrandomized comparison in 90 patients with BPD over a 12-month period. The results of the current study showed reductions in self-harm and improvements in emotional regulation were greater among those receiving DBT than among those receiving MBT. However, this study does not have a follow-up. Experimental studies assessing outcomes beyond 12 months are needed to examine whether these findings represent differences in the clinical effectiveness of these therapies.

Therefore, from a clinical point of view, it is useful to have the possibility of applying both treatment protocols and making decisions about them, taking into account both the clinical situation of the patients and the resources of professionals in a specific clinical context. In this regard, it should be kept in mind that both treatments are quite long (patients usually participate in groups several times: from 6 months to 1.5 years). However, as mentioned above, DBT requires high specialization of the therapist, which is often not possible because of the time and money involved, and standard DBT (the group skills training modules, individual counselling, telephone crisis coaching, and a therapist consultation team) is more difficult to implement in the operating structure of different mental health services, such as public settings. In addition, in our study, dropout rates were similar in the DBT and STEPPS conditions, unlike in other studies where different dropout rates were found (Dixon & Linardon, 2019). Therefore, if a treatment is easier to administer to patients because it entails fewer resources and it is easier to train therapists, these are important factors to consider when making decisions (Bos et al., 2010). However, our results show that DBT obtained better results than STEPPS on some variables. Therefore, the recommendation is that, when the resources for DBT are present in a given clinical context, this treatment should be provided, especially in patients with a worse clinical situation.

Limitations

This study has some limitations. First, it was an open trial that did not offer follow-up data. Second, the assignment of the participants to each treatment condition was not randomized, and so future research should replicate this study using a randomized design. Third, it had a relatively small sample size at the end of treatment. Our sample size increased the possibility of Type II error. Thus, some of the differences that did not reach statistical significance might have been achieved if the sample size had been larger. However, it should also be noted that the sample size is similar to that of other studies on this topic (Linehan et al., 2006; Safer, Robinson, & Jo, 2010), and this work has the advantage of having been carried out in a natural treatment context for patients with BPD, increasing the possibilities of generalizing the results. Finally, although there were no differences in primary and secondary measures between the participants in the two conditions before starting treatment, the DBT group had higher comorbidity and greater severity than the STEPPS group. Although we used severity as a covariate, it is possible that this difference in clinical severity between the two treatment conditions could influence the results at the end of the treatment. Taking all this into account, our results should be considered preliminary data and simply an attempt to compare two different treatments for BPD, thus contributing to the scarce literature on the topic.

Finally, other psychological interventions have been proposed for the treatment of BPD, such as MBT, a psychoanalytically oriented therapeutic approach based on the theory of attachment and the theory of mind (Bateman & Fonagy, 2004), and the "transference-focused psychotherapy," another psychodynamic method based on the relations of the object in the structural organization of the personality (Yeomans, Clarkin, & Kernberg, 2015). In short, there are currently some evidence-based treatments that have been found to contribute to the personal, emotional, social, and physical well-being of patients with BPD. Thus, future research should carry out studies on the effectiveness of DBT versus other psychological interventions with empirical support, in order to find out which intervention is the most effective for participants with BPD. However, it is unusual for the same clinical center to have therapists trained in different orientations. This may be one of the reasons why there are few studies comparing active treatment conditions. Nevertheless, a line of research worth exploring is the personalization of therapy programs. Given that we have several programs with proven efficacy available, it would be important to know which program would work better for a given person.

Conclusion

In summary, the present study confirms that there are treatment programs specifically designed to help BPD patients that have obtained empirical support. Our results support data from the literature showing the effectiveness of these programs in reducing relevant variables, such as BPD symptomatology, suicide risk, or depression (Bateman & Fonagy, 2004; Blum, Bartels, St. John & Pfohl, 2002; Linehan, 1993a, 1993b; Yeomans et al., 2015).

In addition, taking the costs into account, whether in training clinicians or in administering one of the two programs tested in this study in a clinical context, it would be advisable to use STEPPS routinely and, at the same time, if possible, to use DBT for patients with greater severity or clinical comorbidity. In addition, it is necessary to continue to advance in this line of research in order to offer strategies for applying treatments that would represent an improvement for clinicians in terms of the routine application of techniques (for example, treatment sessions whose contents must be repeated in many cases more than once) without affecting their efficacy (Kazdin, 2015; Kazdin & Blase, 2011). To this end, the work being carried out in recent years on the use of the Internet to apply evidence-based psychological treatment protocols (Andrews, Cuijpers, Craske, McEvoy, & Titov, 2010; Karyotaki et al., 2018; Kaltenthaler, Parry, Beverley, & Ferriter, 2008) and carry out assessment strategies (Carlbring et al., 2007; Hedman et al., 2010) can be quite useful. Undoubtedly, new treatment and assessment developments based on the use of information and communication technologies can significantly improve the field of clinical psychology and reduce the burden associated with suffering from a mental disorder.

In this study, we compared the differential effectiveness of two specific psychotherapies for BPD, and we found that both DBT and STEPPS are effective, with DBT being more effective for the behavioral symptoms of BPD.

REFERENCES

American Psychiatric Association. (2000). *Diagnostic and statistical manual of mental disorders* (4th ed., text rev.). Washington, DC: Author.

American Psychiatric Association. (2013). *Diagnostic and statistical manual of mental disorders* (5th ed). Washington, DC: Author.

Andreasson, K., Krogh, J., Wenneberg, C., Jessen, H. K., Krakauer, K., Gluud, C., . . . Nordentoft, M. (2016). Effectiveness of dialectical behavior therapy versus collaborative assessment and management of suicidality treatment for reduction of self-harm in adults with borderline personality traits and disorder—A randomized observer-blinded clinical trial. *Depression and Anxiety*, 33(6), 520–530. https://doi.org/10.1002/da.22472

Andrews, G., Cuijpers, P., Craske, M., McEvoy, P., & Titov, N. (2010). Computer therapy for the anxiety and depressive disorders is effective, acceptable and practical health care: A meta-analysis. *PLoS One*, 5(10), e13196. https://doi.org/10.1371/journal.pone.0013196

Bateman, A., & Fonagy, P. (2004). *Psychotherapy for borderline personality disorder: Mentalization-based treatment*. Oxford, UK: Oxford University Press

Beck, A. T., Steer, R. A., & Brown, G. K. (1996). *Manual for the Beck Depression Inventory-II* (2nd ed.). San Antonio, TX: Psychological Corporation.

Belloch, A., & Fernández Álvarez, H. (2002). *Trastornos de la personalidad* [Personality disorders]. Madrid, Spain: Síntesis.

Barnicot, K., & Crawford, M. (2019). Dialectical behaviour therapy v. mentalisation-based therapy for borderline personality disorder. *Psychological Medicine*, 49, 2060–2068. https://doi.org/10.1017/S0033291718002878

Black, D. W., Blum, N., McCormick, B., & Allen, J. (2013). Systems Training for Emotional Predictability and Problem Solving (STEPPS) group treatment for offenders with borderline personality disorder. *Journal of Nervous and Mental Disease*, 201, 124–129. https://doi.org/10.1097/NMD.0b013e31827f6435

Blum, N., Bartels, N., St. John, D., & Pfohl, B. (2002). *STEPPS: Systems Training for Emotional Predictability and Problem Solving: Group treatment for borderline personality disorder*. Coralville, IA: Blum's Books.

Blum, N., Pfohl, B., John, D. S., Monahan, P., & Black, D. W. (2002). STEPPS: A cognitive-behavioral systems-based group treatment for outpatients with borderline personality disorder—A preliminary report. *Comprehensive Psychiatry*, 43, 301–310. https://doi.org/10.1053/comp.2002.33497

Blum, N., St John, D., Pfohl, B., Stuart, S., McCormick, B., Allen, J., & Black, D. W. (2008). Systems Training for Emotional Predictability and Problem Solving (STEPPS) for outpatients with borderline personality disorder: A randomized controlled trial and 1-year follow-up. *American Journal of Psychiatry*, 165, 468–478. https://doi.org/10.1176/appi.ajp.2007.07071079

Bohus, M., Dyer, A. S., Priebe, K., Krüger, A., Kleindienst, N., Schmahl, C., . . . Steil, R. (2013). Dialectical behaviour therapy for post-traumatic stress disorder after childhood sexual abuse in patients with and without borderline personality disorder: A randomised controlled trial. *Psychotherapy and Psychosomatics, 82*(4), 221–233. https://doi.org/10.1159/000348451

Bohus, M., Kleindienst, N., Limberger, M. F., Stieglitz, R. D., Domsalla, M., Chapman, A. L., ... Wolf, M. (2008). The short version of the Borderline Symptom List (BSL-23): Development and initial data on psychometric properties. *Psychopathology, 42*, 32–39. https://doi.org/10.1159/000173701

Bos, E. H., van Wel, E. B., Appelo, M. T., & Verbraak, M. J. P. M. (2010). A randomized controlled trial of a Dutch version of systems training for emotional predictability and problem solving for borderline personality disorder. *Journal of Nervous and Mental Disease, 198*, 299–304. https://doi.org/10.1097/NMD.0b013e3181d619cf

Burckhardt, R., Manicavasagar, V., Shaw, F., Fogarty, A., Batterham, P. J., Dobinson, K., & Karpin, I. (2018). Preventing mental health symptoms in adolescents using dialectical behaviour therapy skills group: A feasibility study. *International Journal of Adolescence and Youth, 23*, 70–85. https://doi.org/10.1080/02673843.2017.1292927

Carlson, E. B., & Putnam, F. W. (1993). An update on the dissociative experiences scale. *Dissociation: Progress in the Dissociative Disorders, 6*(1), 16–27.

Carlbring, P., Brunt, S., Bohman, S., Austin, D., Richards, J., Öst, L.-G., & Andersson, G. (2007). Internet vs. paper and pencil administration of questionnaires commonly used in panic/agoraphobia research. *Computers in Human Behavior, 23*(3), 1421–1434. https://doi.org/10.1016/j.chb.2005.05.002

Cristea, I. A., Gentili, C., Cotet, C. D., Palomba, D., Barbui, C., & Cuijpers, P. (2017). Efficacy of psychotherapies for borderline personality disorder: A systematic review and meta-analysis. *JAMA Psychiatry, 74*(4), 319–328. https://doi.org/10.1001/jamapsychiatry.2016.4287

DeCou, C., Comtois, K., & Landes, S. (2019). Dialectical behavior therapy is effective for the treatment of suicidal behavior: A meta-analysis. *Behavior Therapy, 50*(1), 60–72. https://doi.org/10.1016/j.beth.2018.03.009

Dixon, L. J., & Linardon, J. (2019). A systematic review and meta-analysis of dropout rates from dialectical behaviour therapy in randomized controlled trials. *Cognitive Behaviour Therapy*. Advance online publication. https://doi.org/10.1080/16506073.2019.1620324

Fitzpatrick, S., Wagner, A. C., & Monson, C. M. (2019). Optimizing borderline personality disorder treatment by incorporating significant others: A review and synthesis. *Personality Disorders: Theory, Research, and Treatment, 10*(4), 297–308. https://doi.org/10.1037/per0000328

George, D., & Mallery, P. (2003). *SPSS for windows step by step: A simple guide and reference* (4th ed). Boston, MA: Allyn and Bacon.

González-Robles, A., Mira, A., Miguel, C., Molinari, G., Díaz-García, A., García-Palacios, A., ... Botella, C. (2018). A brief online transdiagnostic measure: Psychometric properties of the Overall Anxiety Severity and Impairment Scale (OASIS) among Spanish patients with emotional disorders. *PLoS One, 13*(11), e0206516.

Gratz, K. L., & Roemer, L. (2004). Multidimensional assessment of emotion regulation and dysregulation: Development, factor structure, and initial validation of the difficulties in emotion regulation scale. *Journal of Psychopathology and Behavioral Assessment, 26*(1), 41–54. https://doi.org/10.1023/B:JOBA.0000007455.08539.94

Harned, M., Korslund, K., & Linehan, M. (2014). A pilot randomized controlled trial of dialectical behavior therapy with and without the dialectical behavior therapy prolonged exposure protocol for suicidal and self-injuring women with borderline personality disorder and PTSD. *Behaviour Research and Therapy, 55*, 7–17. https://doi.org/10.1016/j.brat.2014.01.008

Harvey, R., Black, D. W., & Blum, N. (2010). Systems training for emotional predictability and problem solving (STEPPS) in the United Kingdom: A preliminary report. *Journal of Contemporary Psychotherapy, 40*, 225–232. https://doi.org/10.1007/s10879-010-9150-4

Hedman, E., Ljótsson, B., Rück, C., Furmark, T., Carlbring, P., Lindefors, N., & Andersson, G. (2010). Internet administration of self-report measures commonly used in research on social anxiety disorder: A psychometric evaluation. *Computers in Human Behavior, 26*, 736–740. https://doi.org/10.1016/j.chb.2010.01.010

Hervás, G., & Jódar, R. (2008). The Spanish version of the Difficulties in Emotion Regulation Scale. *Clínica y Salud, 19*(2), 139–156.

Hill, D., Craighead, L., & Safer, D. (2011). Appetite-focused dialectical behavior therapy for the treatment of binge eating with purging: A preliminary trial. *International Journal of Eating Disorders, 44*(3), 249–261. https://doi.org/10.1002/eat.20812

Icaran, E., Colom, R., & Orengo-García, F. (1996). Experiencias disociativas: Una escala de medida [Dissociative experiences: A measurement scale]. *Anuario de Psicología, 70*, 69–84.

Jones, S. H., Thornicroft, G., Coffey, M., & Dunn, G. (1995). A brief mental health outcome scale-reliability and validity of the Global Assessment of Functioning (GAF). *British*

Journal of Psychiatry, 166(5), 654–659. https://doi.org/10.1192/bjp.166.5.654

Kaltenthaler, E., Parry, G., Beverley, C., & Ferriter, M. (2008). Computerised cognitive-behavioural therapy for depression: Systematic review. *British Journal of Psychiatry, 193*(3), 181–184. https://doi.org/10.1192/bjp.bp.106.025981

Karyotaki, E., Kemmeren, L., Riper, H., Twisk, J., Hoogendoorn, A., & Kleiboer, A., . . . Cuijpers, P. (2018). Is self-guided internet-based cognitive behavioural therapy (iCBT) harmful? An individual participant data meta-analysis. *Psychological Medicine, 48*(15), 2456–2466. https://doi.org/10.1017/s0033291718000648

Kazdin, A., & Blase, S. (2011). Rebooting psychotherapy research and practice to reduce the burden of mental illness. *Perspectives on Psychological Science, 6*(1), 21–37. https://doi.org/10.1177/1745691610393527

Kazdin, A. E. (2015). Technology-based interventions and reducing the burdens of mental illness: Perspectives and comments on the special series. *Cognitive and Behavioral Practice, 22*(3), 359–366. https://doi.org/10.1016/J.CBPRA.2015.04.004

Landes, S. J., Chalker, S. A., & Comtois, K. A. (2016). Predicting dropout in outpatient dialectical behavior therapy with patients with borderline personality disorder receiving psychiatric disability. *Borderline Personality Disorder and Emotion Dysregulation, 3*(1), 9. https://doi.org/10.1186/s40479-016-0043-3

Linardon, J., Fairburn, C., Fitzsimmons-Craft, E., Wilfley, D., & Brennan, L. (2017). The empirical status of the third-wave behaviour therapies for the treatment of eating disorders: A systematic review. *Clinical Psychology Review, 58*, 125–140. https://doi.org/10.1016/j.cpr.2017.10.005

Linardon, J., Gleeson, J., Yap, K., Murphy, K., & Brennan, L. (2019). Meta-analysis of the effects of third-wave behavioural interventions on disordered eating and body image concerns: Implications for eating disorder prevention. *Cognitive Behaviour Therapy, 48*(1), 15–38. https://doi.org/10.1080/16506073.2018.1517389

Linehan, M. M. (1993a). *Cognitive-behavioral treatment of borderline personality disorder.* New York, NY: Guilford Press

Linehan, M. M. (1993b). *Skills training manual for treating borderline personality disorder.* New York, NY: Guilford Press.

Linehan, M. M. (2014). *DBT skills training manual* (2nd ed.). New York, NY: Guilford Press.

Linehan, M. M., Armstrong, H. E., Suarez, A., Allmon, D., & Heard, H. L. (1991). Cognitive-behavioral treatment of chronically parasuicidal borderline patients. *Archives of General Psychiatry, 48*(12), 1060–1064. https://doi.org/10.1001/archpsyc1991.01810360024003

Linehan, M. M., Comtois, K. A., Murray, A. M., Brown, M. Z., Gallop, R. J., & Heard, H. L., . . . Lindenboim, M. (2006). Two-year randomized controlled trial and follow-up of dialectical behavior therapy vs therapy by experts for suicidal behaviors and borderline personality disorder. *Archives of General Psychiatry, 63*(7), 757–766. https://doi.org/10.1001/archpsyc.63.7.757

Linehan, M. M., Goodstein, J. L., Nielsen, S. L., & Chiles, J. A. (1983). Reasons for staying alive when you are thinking of killing yourself: The Reasons for Living Inventory. *Journal of Consulting and Clinical Psychology, 51*(2), 276–286. https://doi.org/10.1037/0022-006X.51.2.276

McMain, S. F., Guimond, T., Barnhart, R., Habinski, L., & Streiner, D. L. (2017). A randomized trial of brief dialectical behavior therapy skills training in suicidal patients suffering from borderline disorder. *Acta Psychiatrica Scandinavica, 135*(2), 138–148. https://doi.org/10.1111/acps.12664

McMain, S. F., Links, P. S., Gnam, W. H., Guimond, T., Cardish, R. J., Korman, L., & Streiner, D. L. (2009). A randomized trial of dialectical behavior therapy versus general psychiatric management for borderline personality disorder. *American Journal of Psychiatry, 166*(12), 1365–1374. https://doi.org/10.1176/appi.ajp.2009.09010039

Mezzich, J. E., Ruipérez, M. A., Pérez, C., Yoon, G., Liu, J., & Mahmud, S. (2000). The Spanish version of the quality of life index: Presentation and validation. *Journal of Nervous and Mental Disease, 188*(5), 301–305. https://doi.org/10.1097/00005053-200005000-00008

Miguel-Tobal, J., Casado, M., Cano-Vindel, A., & Spielberger, C. (2001). *Inventario de Expresión de la Ira Estado-Rasgo STAXI-2 [State-Trait Anger Expression Inventory STAXI-2].* Madrid, Spain: TEA Ediciones.

Neacsiu, A. D., Lungu, A., Harned, M. S., Rizvi, S. L., & Linehan, M. M. (2014). Impact of dialectical behavior therapy versus community treatment by experts on emotional experience, expression, and acceptance in borderline personality disorder. *Behaviour Research and Therapy, 53*, 47–54. https://doi.org/10.1016/j.brat.2013.12.004

Norman, S., Hami Cissell, S., Means-Christensen, A., & Stein, M. (2006). Development and validation of an Overall Anxiety Severity and Impairment Scale (OASIS). *Depression and Anxiety, 23*(4), 245–249. https://doi.org/10.1002/da.20182

Oquendo, M. A., Baca-Garcia, E., Graver, R., Morales, M., Montalvan, V., & Mann, J. J. (2000). Spanish adaptation of the Reasons for Living Inventory. *Hispanic Journal of Behavioral Sciences, 22*(3), 369–381. https://doi.org/10.1177/0739986300223006

Oquendo, M. A., Baca-Garcia, E., Graver, R., Morales, M., Montalvan, V., & Mann, J. (2001). Spanish adaptation of the Barratt Impulsiveness Scale (BIS-11). *European Journal of Psychiatry, 15*(3), 147–155.

Pasieczny, N., & Connor, J. (2011). The effectiveness of dialectical behaviour therapy in routine public mental health settings: An Australian controlled trial. *Behaviour Research and Therapy, 49*(1), 4–10. https://doi.org/10.1016/j.brat.2010.09.006

Patton, J. H., Stanford, M. S., & Barratt, E. S. (1995). Factor structure of the Barratt Impulsiveness Scale. *Journal of Clinical Psychology, 51*(6), 768–774. https://doi.org/10.1002/1097-4679(199511)51:6<768::aid-jclp2270510607>3.0.co;2-1

Plutchik, R., Van Praag, H., Conte, H. R., & Picard, S. (1989). Correlates of suicide and violence risk, I: The suicide risk measure. *Comprehensive Psychiatry, 30*, 296–302. https://doi.org/10.1016/0010-440X(89)90053-9

Priebe, S., Bhatti, N., Barnicot, K., Bremner, S., Gaglia, A., Katsakou, C., . . . Zinkler, M. (2012). Effectiveness and cost-effectiveness of dialectical behaviour therapy for self-harming patients with personality disorder: A pragmatic randomised controlled trial. *Psychotherapy and Psychosomatics, 81*(6), 356–365. https://doi.org/10.1159/000338897

Reimann, G., Weisscher, N., Goossens, P. J., Draijer, N., Apenhorst-Hol, M., & Kulpa, R. W. (2014). The addition of STEPPS in the treatment of patients with bipolar disorder and comorbid borderline personality features: A protocol for a randomized control trial. *BMC Psychiatry, 14*, 172. https://doi.org/10.1186/1471-244X-14-172

Rubio, G., Montero, I., Jáuregui, J., Villanueva, R., Casado, M. A., Marin, J. J., & Santo-Domingo, J. (1998). Assessing the validity of the Plutchik Suicide Risk Scale in a sample of Spanish population. *Archivos de Neurobiología, 61*, 149–158.

Safer, D., Robinson, A., & Jo, B. (2010). Outcome from a randomized controlled trial of group therapy for binge eating disorder: Comparing dialectical behavior therapy adapted for binge eating to an active comparison group therapy. *Behavior Therapy, 41*(1), 106–120. https://doi.org/10.1016/j.beth.2010.04.001

Safer, D., Telch, C., & Agras, W. (2001). Dialectical behavior therapy for bulimia nervosa. *American Journal of Psychiatry, 158*(4), 632–634. https://doi.org/10.1176/appi.ajp.158.4.632

Sanz, J., Perdigón, A. L., & Vazquez, C. (2003). Adaptación española del Inventario para la Depresión de Beck-II (BDI-II): 2. Propiedades psicométricas en población general [Spanish adaptation of the Beck Depression Inventory II (BDI-II): 2. Psychometric properties in the general population]. *Clínica y Salud, 14*(3), 249–280.

Soler, J., Vega, D., Feliu-Soler, A., Trujols, J., Soto, Á., & Elices, M., . . . Pascual, J. C. (2013). Validation of the Spanish version of the Borderline Symptom List, short form (BSL-23). *BMC Psychiatry, 13*(1), 139. https://doi.org/10.1186/1471-244x-13-139

Spielberger, C. (1999). *State-Trait Anger Expression Inventory-2: Professional manual*. Lutz, FL: Psychological Assessment Resources.

Spielberger, C., Miguel-Tobal, J., Cano-Vindel, A., & Casado-Morales, M. (2006). *Inventario de expresión de ira estado-rasgo: STAXI-2 2 [State-Trait Anger Expression Inventory; STAXI-2]*. Madrid, Spain: TEA.

Wilks, S. E. (2008). Psychometric evaluation of the shortened resilience scale among Alzheimer's caregivers. *American Journal of Alzheimer's Disease and Other Dementias, 23*(2), 143–149. https://doi.org/10.1111/j.1547-5069.1990.tb00224.x

Yeomans, F., Clarkin, J., & Kernberg, O. (2015). *Transference-focused psychotherapy for borderline personality disorder*. Washington, DC: Author.

Maladaptive Fearlessness: An Examination of the Association Between Subjective Fear Experience and Antisocial Behaviors Linked with Callous Unemotional Traits

Elise M. Cardinale, PhD, Rebecca M. Ryan, PhD, and Abigail A. Marsh, PhD

> The centrality of a fearless temperament as it relates to the construct of psychopathy remains an area of controversy, with some researchers arguing that the relationship between fearless temperament and psychopathy (and associated antisocial behavior) can be explained by shared associations with other core affective and interpersonal traits of psychopathy such as callous-unemotional (CU) traits. The authors investigated real-world subjectively experienced fear in 306 individuals with varying levels of CU traits and antisocial behavior and found that at low levels of subjective fear experience, decreases in subjective fear were associated with greater antisociality. Even after controlling for the positive relationship between CU traits and antisocial behavior, reduced subjectively experienced fear remained a significant predictor of antisocial behavior. These results provide evidence that experienced fear is related to antisocial behavior at lower than average levels of subjectively experienced fear and that this relationship persists after controlling for CU traits.
>
> *Keywords*: fear, callous-unemotional traits, antisocial behavior, emotion, psychopathy

Disproportionate engagement in antisocial and aggressive behavior is closely associated with psychopathic personality traits (Hare & Neumann, 2010; Leistico, Salekin, DeCoster, & Rogers, 2008) and is a central part of most conceptualizations of the construct of psychopathy (Blair, 2005; Cleckley, 1976; Hare, 2006). Interest persists in how callous-unemotional (CU) traits, the core affective and interpersonal deficits characteristic of psychopathy (Frick & Ray, 2015), distinguish individuals with psychopathic traits from other antisocial populations. However, the relative importance of certain affective and interpersonal traits—specifically, a fearless temperament—in predicting antisocial behavior remains an area of controversy (Lilienfeld et al., 2012; Lynam &

From Department of Psychology, Georgetown University, Washington, DC.

Address correspondence to Elise M. Cardinale, Department of Psychology, Georgetown University, 3700 P St. NW, Washington, DC 20057. E-mail: emc62@georgetown.edu

---

Originally published in the *Journal of Personality Disorders*, Volume 35, Supplement A. ©2021 The Guilford Press.

Miller, 2012; Marcus, Fulton, & Edens, 2013; Patrick, Venables, & Drislane, 2013), with some arguing that fearless traits are key developmental drivers in the emergence of psychopathic traits and resulting antisocial behavior (Blair, 2013; Frick & White, 2008; Lykken, 2013; Waller, Shaw, & Hyde, 2017; S. F. White et al., 2016). Others contend that observed low associations between measures of fearless traits and antisocial behaviors provide evidence that, while fearless traits may be associated with the construct of the psychopathic personality, these traits play little to no important role in the emergence of antisocial and aggressive behavior (Miller & Lynam, 2012; Seibert, Miller, Few, Zeichner, & Lynam, 2011). The current study aims to further probe the question of the role of fearless traits in the interpersonal and affective features of psychopathy by investigating the associations among antisocial behavior, CU traits, and ecological experiences of fear in a setting designed to evoke extreme fear.

Psychopathy is typically defined as an aggregation of temperamental and behavioral traits that include a callous disposition, bold and dominant social behavior, disinhibition, and persistent antisociality (Cleckley, 1976; Hare, 2006). This constellation of traits has been consistently and robustly associated with deficits in a wide array of subjective and physiological responses to threat. For example, when presented with threatening stimuli, individuals with psychopathic traits exhibit reductions in fear-potentiated startle responding (Fanti, Panayiotou, Lazarou, Michael, & Georgiou, 2016; Kimonis, Fanti, Goulter, & Hall, 2017; Levenston, Patrick, Bradley, & Lang, 2000), electrodermal reactivity (Hare, 1982; Lorber, 2004; Lykken, 1957; Thomson et al., 2018), and fearful facial expressions (Herpertz et al., 2001). Psychopathic traits also impair avoidance learning (Blair et al., 2004; Lykken, 1957) and Pavlovian fear conditioning (Birbaumer et al., 2005; Flor, Birbaumer, Hermann, Ziegler, & Patrick, 2002; Rothemund et al., 2012). Recent meta-analytic findings also confirm that fearlessness is relevant to many well-validated measures of psychopathy (Lilienfeld et al., 2016).

Fearless traits are central to various theories about why psychopathy and antisocial behavior emerge during development. Lack of negative arousal during transgressions that result in punishment in children with fearless temperaments is believed to prevent the development of guilt and empathy in response to such transgressions and ultimately lead to the development of CU traits and antisocial behavior (Decety, 2010; Frick & Morris, 2004; Kochanska, Gross, Lin, & Nichols, 2002). This may be because impaired fear responding also impairs empathic responding to the fear and distress of others (Cardinale et al., 2018; Marsh, 2018; Marsh & Cardinale, 2012, 2014). The Integrated Emotion Systems model of psychopathy (Blair, 2005, 2013; Blair, Hwang, White, & Meffert, 2016) further proposes that transgressions that cause distress in others come to be regarded as wrong through stimulus-reinforcement learning. These transgressions and their association with the aversive feedback of the distress of the victim result in conditioning of the transgressions themselves as aversive. When this stimulus-reinforcement learning is impaired in individuals with psychopathic traits due to low responsiveness to fear in others, transgressions that cause distress in others fail to be conditioned as aversive and therefore are more likely to occur in individuals with psychopathic traits. Finally, the low arousal theory of aggression (Raine, 1996, 2002) purports that low autonomic arousal, a marker of fearlessness, predisposes individuals to engage in risky antisocial and violent behavior (Raine, 1996). Consistent with this theory, a meta-analysis of 40 papers found the best replicated biological predictor of antisocial behavior to be low resting heart rate (Ortiz & Raine, 2004).

A number of longitudinal studies have also demonstrated a link between impoverished fear responding and antisocial behavior. For example, reduced electrodermal activity during a Pavlonian fear-conditioning paradigm as early as 3 years of age is predictive of aggressive behavior at age 8 (Gao, Raine, Venables, Dawson, & Mednick, 2010) and adult criminal offending at age 23 (Gao, Raine, Venables, Dawson, & Mednick, 2009). Furthermore, observations of fearless temperament at 42 months is predictive of callous-unemotional behaviors at ages 10–12 years old in infants with low levels of positive parenting (Waller et al, 2017). Together, this body of literature suggests that impoverished physiological and subjective fear responses to threats and punishment may represent a neurobehavioral mechanism underlying antisocial behavior in adults with psychopathic traits.

But skepticism persists regarding the relevance of fearless traits as part of the construct of psychopathy, in part due to relatively small within-person associations between fearless-dominant traits and the antisocial behavioral components of psychopathy, including aggression (Lynam & Miller, 2012; Marcus et al., 2013). In a meta-analysis of 61 samples, measurements of fearless dominance showed relatively weak associations with measures of empathy, externalizing behaviors, and aggression compared to other factors of psychopathy (Miller & Lynam, 2012). There are at least two possible explanations for these findings. First, fearless dominance may be an emergent property of core interpersonal and affective traits characteristic of psychopathy, such as callous or uncaring traits. In this case, fearless traits may have little direct effect on the development of antisocial behavior, and they may be less central to the construct of psychopathy than other traits. If this were true, we would expect that any relationship between fearlessness and aggression would be dependent on shared associations with other traits central to psychopathy, such as callous or uncaring traits.

An alternate possibility is that existing measures of fearless-dominant traits may not adequately capture fearless temperamental traits, but rather more diffuse deficits, such as deficits in negative emotionality or in social dominance. Much of the work calling into question the link between fearlessness and the affective and interpersonal features of psychopathy relies on trait measurements of fearlessness rather than on laboratory measures of fear responding. For example, personality assessments of fearlessness in psychopathy focus on the dimension of fearless dominance or boldness. This dimension of psychopathy is particularly characteristic of primary psychopathy and involves traits such as lack of fear, charm, and risk-seeking behaviors (Levenson, Kiehl, & Fitzpatrick, 1995; Lilienfeld & Andrews, 1996). The use of these measures may artificially reduce the apparent association between fearless traits and aggression, in part because these measurements do not assess fearlessness specifically, but rather focus on global assessments of reduced negative emotionality (i.e., neuroticism, internalizing symptoms) and increased positive emotionality (i.e., extraversion, novelty seeking). Direct assessments of experiences of fear, particularly in ecologically valid settings, may yield more robust associations between psychopathy, fearless traits, and antisocial behaviors. No prior study has examined how subjective experiences of ecologically induced fear are associated with psychopathy or antisocial behaviors, due in part to ethical limitations on the nature of emotional experiences that can be induced in the laboratory (e.g., research participants cannot be exposed to genuine danger or risk that would elicit highly variable levels of fear). Thus, there remains a need for research examining subjectively experienced ecologically valid fear and its associations with antisociality and the core affective and interpersonal traits associated with psychopathy (CU traits).

The current study aimed to fill this gap by investigating the relationships among ecologically evoked fear experiences, CU traits, and antisocial behavior. Consistent with the large body of work reviewed above linking psychopathic traits with reduced responses to fear (Fanti et al., 2016; Hare, 1982; Herpertz et al., 2001; Kimonis et al., 2017; Levenston et al., 2000; Lorber, 2004; Lykken, 1957; Thomson et al., 2018), we predicted that fearlessness, as measured by relatively low self-reported fear in a highly fear-eliciting environment, would be related to characteristic components of the psychopathic personality. In addition, bolstered by evidence that low autonomic arousal robustly relates to engagement in antisocial behaviors (Ortiz & Raine, 2004), we predicted that fearlessness would predict aggressive behavior above and beyond other measurements of the affective and interpersonal traits associated with psychopathy, such as callous traits.

To test these hypotheses, we collected data from a moderately large community sample of adults recruited at a nationally ranked seasonal haunted attraction in the Washington, DC, region called Markoff's Haunted Forest. Within this setting, we collected measurements of robust and ecological subjective experiences of amusement, anger, disgust, fear, and sadness. We then assessed the relationship between these subjectively experienced emotions and scores on the Inventory of Callous and Unemotional Traits (ICU) as well as self-reported instances of antisocial behaviors. We predicted that respondents who reported experiencing lower levels of subjective fear in a highly fear-evoking context would report higher CU traits and antisocial behavior. Furthermore, we expected that including a measure of fearlessness would strengthen the predictive power of a model predicting antisocial behavior from CU traits. Finally, we hypothesized that the subjective experience of fear would be more strongly associated with antisocial behavior than more general measurements of impoverished negative emotionality such as the unemotional subscale of the ICU.

METHODS

Participants

Following approval from the Georgetown University Institutional Review Board, 306 community sample participants, ages 18 to 59 ($M = 30.93$, $SD = 8.89$), completed our study. Of these, 163 participants identified as male and 135 as female, and 8 participants declined to indicate their gender. Participants were recruited from a nationally ranked seasonal haunted attraction in

Poolesville, Maryland. Researchers approached individuals immediately after they exited the Haunted Forest in order to complete the study as soon after they left the attraction as possible (latency $M = 9.89$ min, $SD = 13.24$ min). In the Forest, participants complete a dark self-guided walk at night through one of two trails located at Calleva Farm. Each trail takes approximately 20 minutes to complete and requires passing through approximately 13 immersive scenes, during which patrons walk through sites such as graveyards, swamps, and a tattered circus tent while interacting with hired actors playing zombies, clowns, and chainsaw-wielding murderers (Joynt, 2012). Aspects of these settings are designed to elicit a range of strong emotions, including anger, disgust, fear, and amusement.

Measures

Subjective Emotional Experience Questionnaire. The Subjective Emotional Experience Questionnaire (Marsh et al., 2011) consisted of questions inquiring about respondents' emotional experiences in the Forest—including experiences of five basic emotions: anger, disgust, fear, happiness, and sadness. Participants indicated their subjective experience of each of the five emotions using a visual analog scale, drawing a vertical mark on a horizontal line anchored on the left by "none at all" and on the right by "a lot." Responses were scored as the distance in millimeters from the left end of the line, such that higher values correspond with greater levels of subjectively experienced emotion.

In addition, participants reported variables relevant to sympathetic and parasympathetic nervous system activity (Marsh et al., 2011; Scherer & Wallbott, 1994). Items on this scale include statements such as "My body feels tense" and "My heart is beating faster." Participants were instructed to rate the degree to which they felt each of the 12 body sensations using 7-point scales. The composite index of sympathetic activation consists of the average of items measuring breathing changes, increases in heart rate, muscle tension, increases in energy, and perspiration, and the composite index of parasympathetic activation consists of the average of items measuring stomach trouble, body relaxation, and lump in throat.

Finally, we obtained ratings of general fearfulness in daily life using three questions: "Please rate how easy or hard it is for you to remember times you have felt afraid in the past" (1 = *Very hard*, 7 = *Very easy*), "Compared to most people, how often do you usually feel afraid?" (1 = *Not very often*, 7 = *Very often*), and "Compared to most people, how strongly do you usually feel afraid?" (1 = *Not very strongly*, 7 = *Very strongly*). We observed the full range of responses within our sample for all three general fearfulness items: how often do you feel fear? ($M = 3.17$, $SD = 1.54$), how strongly do you feel fear? ($M = 3.51$, $SD = 1.63$), and how easy is it to remember past fear? ($M = 4.69$, $SD = 1.71$), suggesting that our sample did not consist of uniformly fearless respondents.

Inventory of Callous and Unemotional Traits. The Inventory of Callous and Unemotional Traits (ICU) is a 24-item self-report assessment of the core affective and interpersonal characteristics of psychopathy and includes items associated with three subscales: callous, unemotional, and uncaring (Kimonis et al., 2008). Participants rated each item using a 4-point response scale (0 = *not true at all*, 3 = *definitely true*). The scale was originally developed for use with children and adolescents, but it shows comparable properties in adults (Byrd, Kahn, & Pardini, 2013; Drislane, Patrick, & Arsal, 2014; Drislane et al., 2015; Fix & Fix, 2015; Kimonis, Branch, Hagman, Graham, & Miller, 2013; Schenk, Ragatz, & Fremouw, 2012; Stoeber, 2015; B. A. White, Gordon, & Guerra, 2015; A. C. White & Miller, 2014). Scores for the total ICU scale and all three subscales were calculated for each of the participants (Table 1). Total ICU scores ranged from 0 to 43 ($M = 17.41$, $SD = 8.71$). Reliability of the total scale was $\alpha = .81$. Examined separately, the unemotional, callous, and uncaring subscales had reliabilities of $\alpha = .77$, $.74$, and $.69$, respectively.

Self-Reported Antisocial Behavior. We used a brief 2-item scale to assess serious lifetime antisocial behaviors. Participants reported the number of physical fights they had been in and the total number of times they had been arrested. Participants' reported numbers of physical fights ranged from 0 to 200 ($M = 2.80$, $SD = 13.52$), and arrests ranged from 0 to 10 ($M = 0.29$, $SD = 0.94$). We summed the two items to create a composite antisociality

TABLE 1. Descriptive Statistics for All Experimental Scales

	Range	Mean (*SD*)	Skewness	Kurtosis
ICU				
Total Score	0–43	17.41 (8.71)	0.67	3.20
Unemotional	0–18	5.99 (3.33)	1.31	4.40
Callous	0–24	5.98 (4.64)	1.31	4.40
Uncaring	0–19	5.51 (3.69)	0.84	3.49
Emotional Experience				
Amusement	0–101	75.57 (19.11)	−1.52	5.48
Anger	0–96	9.14 (15.81)	3.43	16.20
Disgust	0–92	11.27 (15.86)	2.48	10.25
Fear	0–100	54.30 (27.62)	−0.32	2.00
Sadness	0–100	8.04 (15.67)	3.83	19.16
General Fear Experience				
How easy to remember fear in the past	1–7	4.69 (1.71)	−0.34	2.91
How often do you feel afraid	1–7	3.17 (1.54)	0.51	2.34
How strongly do you feel fear	1–7	3.51 (1.62)	0.28	2.64
Nervous System Activity				
Parasympathetic activity	1–6	2.25 (0.86)	0.73	3.98
Sympathetic activity	1–7	3.57 (1.39)	0.10	2.17
Serious Lifetime Antisociality				
Physical fights	0–200	2.80 (13.52)	12.26	168.83
Arrests	0–10	0.29 (0.94)	5.79	47.80
Antisociality Index	0–204.5	3.08 (13.85)	12.09	166.01

Note. ICU = Inventory of Callous Unemotional Traits.

index for each participant that reflected the count of both self-reported physical fights and arrests ($M = 3.075$, $SD = 13.85$). For purposes of validation, a subset of the participants ($n = 94$) also completed the Reactive and Proactive Aggression Questionnaire (RPQ; Raine et al., 2006). We calculated the total RPQ ($M = 10.43$, $SD = 7.39$), reactive aggression ($M = 7.17$, $SD = 4.23$), and proactive aggression ($M = 3.26$, $SD = 4.03$) scores. The antisociality index was significantly associated with overall RPQ scores, IRR = 1.09 (95% CI [1.02, 1.15]), $z(94) = 2.76$, $p = .01$, and was more strongly associated with proactive aggression, IRR = 1.12 (95% CI [1.01, 1.25]), $z(94) = 2.20$, $p = .03$, than reactive aggression, IRR = 1.05 (95% CI [0.92, 1.20]), $z(94) = 0.46$, $p = .46$.

Analytic Strategy

Three separate researchers entered all survey data separately. Data entry was then evaluated using the program DiffMerge in order to ensure consistent entry of all raw data from paper-pencil to digital format. Given the nonnormality of many of the variables of interest (Table 1), all analyses were repeated using Huber-White corrected standard errors to be robust against heteroskedasticity. All analyses predicting antisociality were repeated using negative binomial regressions in order to accommodate both the over dispersion and count nature of the dependent variable. Because of a substantial number of 0 values in the antisociality index, for each model in our results, we report the results of a Vuong test, which was used to determine whether a zero-inflated model was a significantly better fit for the data (Long & Freese, 2006). If significant, models were rerun as a zero-inflated negative binomial. In our sample, both age and gender were associated with all three of our variables of interest (reported subjective fear experience, ICU scores, and antisociality). Therefore, we repeated all analyses with these two variables entered as covariates. Because a linear increase in age is not hypothesized to be causally related to increases in instances of antisocial behavior, for analyses examining antisociality, age effects are best modeled as an exposure variable such that increases in age reflect increasing opportunity to engage in antisocial behavior. Akaike's information criteria (AIC) and Bayesian information criteria (BIC) were used as indices for model comparison where smaller values indicate a better model fit.

RESULTS

Subjective Experience of Emotion

Emotional experience in Markoff's Haunted Forest was assessed by examining both self-reported subjective experiences of emotion and of parasympathetic and sympathetic nervous system activation. Across all participants, subjective experiences of all emotions were endorsed (e.g., indicated levels > 0), indicating that some degree of each of the five surveyed emotions was subjectively experienced across participants. On average, participants reported the highest levels of amusement ($M = 75.57$, $SD = 19.11$) and fear ($M = 54.30$, $SD = 27.62$), followed by disgust ($M = 11.27$, $SD = 15.86$), anger ($M = 9.14$, $SD = 15.81$), and sadness ($M = 8.04$, $SD = 15.67$). Reports of autonomic activation ranged from 1 to 7 for sympathetic activation ($M = 3.57, SD = 1.39$) and from 1 to 6 for parasympathetic activation ($M = 2.25, SD = 0.86$) (Table 1). Self-reported parasympathetic activation was positively associated with the subjective experiences of anger, disgust, and sadness. Self-reported sympathetic activation was positively associated with the subject experiences of anger, disgust, fear, and sadness (Table 2).

To assess the association between self-reported subjective experiences of fear in Markoff's Haunted Forest and trait-level fear, we examined bivariate correlations between subjectively experienced fear and the three trait-level fearfulness items. Responses to how often, $r = .37, p < .001$, and how strongly, $r = .33, p < .001$, individuals reported feeling fear generally were significantly associated with reported experiences of fear in the Forest. The third item, reported ease of remembering past fear, was marginally correlated with reports of fear, $r = .11, p = .06$.

We repeated all analyses with age and gender included as covariates. Results of these regression analyses, with robust standard errors, confirmed all of the associations found using bivariate correlational analyses, with one exception, which was that sympathetic activation and subjectively experienced sadness were associated only at a trend level, $b = .01, t(275) = 1.81, p = .07$.

Serious Lifetime Antisocial Behavior

Associations With Subjective Experience of Emotion. Bivariate correlations between each subjectively experienced emotion in the Forest and serious lifetime antisociality were calculated. Only experienced fear was associated with serious lifetime antisociality, $r = -.19, p = .002$. However, inspection of the data indicated a nonlinear relationship between emotion experience and antisocial

TABLE 2. Bivariate Correlations Between Emotion Experience at Markoff's Haunted Forest and Inventory of Callous Unemotional Traits (ICU)

	1	2	3	4	5	6	7	8	9	10	11	12
1. Amusement	—											
2. Anger	−.07	—										
3. Disgust	−.15*	.60**	—									
4. Fear	.09	.25**	.21**	—								
5. Sadness	−.01	.40**	.51**	.08	—							
6. Parasympathetic	−.07	.29**	.25**	−.02	.21**	—						
7. Sympathetic	−.00	.24**	.30**	.59**	.13*	.15*	—					
8. Total ICU	−.16**	.14*	.06	−.12*	.04	.12	−.04	—				
9. Unemotional	−.19**	−.03	−.03	−.15*	−.03	.03	−.08	.66**	—			
10. Callous	−.10	.19**	.09	−.10	.07	.16*	−.01	.81**	.29**	—		
11. Uncaring	−.14*	.10	.04	−.02	.02	.06	−.03	.75**	.30**	.39**	—	
12. Antisociality	.10	−.02	−.05	−.19*	.04	.06	−.13*	.08	−.01	.13*	.03	—
13. Age	.16*	−.15*	.21**	−.11	−.12*	−.06	−.14*	−.08	−.09	−.07	−.01	.25

Note: *$p < .05$. **$p < .001$.

behavior. We repeated our analyses using a negative binomial regression with robust standard errors, gender entered as a covariate, and age entered as an exposure variable. Results of separate negative binomial regressions predicting antisociality revealed that none of the subjectively reported emotions were linearly associated with self-reported antisociality. However, a significant quadratic relationship, IRR = 1.0004, z = 2.41, p = .02, between fear experience and antisociality was identified such that at low levels of fear (scores lower than 56.32)the negative relationship between subjectively experienced fear and serious lifetime antisociality was significant, IRR = 0.95, z = –2.62, p = .01, whereas at higher levels of fear, no relationship between experienced fear and antisociality emerged (Figure 1). No other emotion showed a significant quadratic relationship with antisocial behavior.

Associations With CU Traits. To assess the relationship between serious lifetime antisociality and CU traits, we first examined bivariate correlations between total and subscale scores on the ICU and serious lifetime antisociality. Only scores on the callous subscale were significantly associated with antisociality, r = .13 p = .03. We next conducted separate negative binomial regression with robust standard errors for total ICU scores and each of the subscales predicting antisociality with gender as a covariate and age entered as an exposure variable. Results confirmed that antisociality was positively

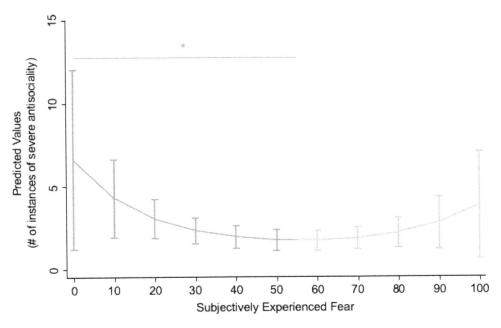

FIGURE 1. Predicted Margins for the Quadratic Effect Between Subjectively Experienced Fear and Severe Lifetime Antisociality. The association between subjectively experienced fear and serious lifetime antisociality is significant at scores lower than 56.32. Error bars represent the 95% confidence interval.

associated with scores on the callous subscale, IRR = 1.09, z = 3.49, p < .001. In addition, total scores on the ICU were significantly associated with increased levels of antisociality, IRR = 1.04, z = 2.77, p = .01. Scores on neither the unemotional subscale, IRR = 1.01, z = 0.13, p = .89, nor the uncaring subscale, IRR = 1.04, z = 1.46, p = .15, were significantly associated with serious lifetime antisociality. The results of a negative binomial regression in which all three subscales were entered as predictors of antisocial behavior also found callousness to be the only significant predictor of antisocial behavior, IRR = 1.10, $z(278)$ = 3.53, p < .001, even after controlling for unemotional and uncaring subscale scores.

Subjective Experience of Emotion and Callous-Unemotional Traits

To assess the relationship between subjectively experienced emotions and CU traits, we first calculated bivariate correlations between ICU total scores and subjective emotional experiences in the Forest. Total ICU scores were negatively associated with both the intensity of experienced amusement, r = −.16 p = .01, and fear, r = −.12 p = .04, and positively associated with the intensity of experienced anger, r = .14 p = .02 (Table 2). Examination of the three subscales of the ICU showed that scores on the unemotional subscale were negatively associated with subjectively experienced amusement, r = −.16, p = .01, and fear, r = −.11, p = .04, whereas scores on the callous subscale were positively associated with subjectively experienced anger only, r = .19, p = .001. Scores on the uncaring subscale were not significantly associated with any of the subjectively experienced emotions. We again conducted regression analyses with robust standard errors and age and gender entered as covariates. We entered subjective emotional experiences into separate regression analyses predicting total ICU scores. Results revealed that only subjectively experienced amusement, b = −.09, $t(280)$ = −3.09, p = .002, and anger, b = .082, $t(272)$ = 2.03, p = .04, were linearly related to total scores on the ICU. Relationships between subjectively experienced emotions and ICU subscale scores were also examined through separate regression analyses, with robust errors and age and gender entered as covariates. Results of regression analyses were consistent with the results of all bivariate correlation with one exception: Uncaring subscale scores showed a marginally significant relationship with subjectively experienced fear, b = −.025, $t(280)$ = −1.93, p = .06.

Because a quadratic relationship between subjectively experienced fear and serious lifetime antisociality was observed, we tested for a quadratic relationship between each subjectively experienced emotion and ICU scores, with age and gender as covariates and robust standard errors. Subjectively experienced fear showed a significant quadratic relationship with total ICU scores, b = .002, $t(281)$ = 2.44, p = .02, such that only at low levels of fear experience (scores lower than 59.06), was fear negatively associated with increased total ICU scores, b = −.21, $t(281)$ = −2.70, p = .01 (Figure 2). Experienced fear also showed a significant quadratic relationship with callous subscale scores, b = .001, $t(281)$ = 2.53, p = .01, such that at low levels of fear experience (scores lower than 56.79), subjectively experienced fear was

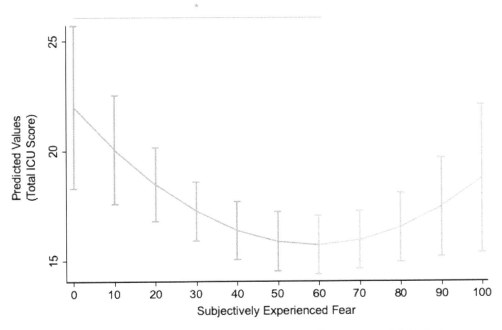

FIGURE 2. Predicted Margins for the Quadratic Effect Between Subjectively Experienced Fear and Total ICU Score. The association between subjectively experienced fear and serious lifetime antisociality is significant at scores lower than 59.06. Error bars represent the 95% confidence interval.

negatively associated with increased scores on the callous subscale, b = −.12, $t(281) = -2.59$, $p = .01$. No other quadratic relationships were observed between subjectively experienced emotions and total ICU or subscale scores.

Fear, CU Traits, and Antisocial Behavior

Total ICU Scores. We next aimed to identify whether subjectively experienced fear and ICU scores both remain significant predictors of severe lifetime antisociality after controlling for shared variance between these two variables. Therefore, we conducted a negative binomial regression with antisociality regressed on total ICU scores and fear experience. We entered both the linear and quadratic terms for fear into this regression model, as well as gender as a covariate and age as an exposure variable. We again used robust standard errors. Results showed that both total scores on the ICU, IRR = 1.03, $z = 2.02$, $p = .04$, and fear experience were significantly associated with serious lifetime antisociality. Fear experience again had a significant quadratic relationship, IRR = 1.0004, $z = 2.03$, $p = .04$, such that at low levels of fear experience (scores lower than 56.39), the negative relationship between subjectively experienced fear and antisociality was significant, IRR = 0.96, $z = -2.20$, $p = .03$. This regression model predicting antisociality with both total ICU scores and subjectively experienced fear fit the data better, AIC = 995.54, BIC = 1017.18, than a model including only total scores on the ICU, AIC = 1028.46, BIC = 1042.88. Lastly, we examined the interaction between total ICU scores and subjectively experienced fear in the prediction of antisociality. In this last model, we regressed antisociality on subjectively experienced fear, total ICU scores, and gender, with age as an exposure variable, and robust standard errors. Results revealed no significant interaction between total scores on the ICU and subjectively experienced fear on antisociality.

Callous Subscale Scores. We repeated these analyses with scores on the callous subscale and fear together predicting antisocial behavior. We first ran a negative binomial regression with scores on the callous subscale of the ICU and subjective fear experience as predictors of antisociality with gender entered as a covariate and age entered as an exposure variable. Results revealed that scores on the callous subscale remained a significant predictor of antisociality, IRR = 1.08, $z = 2.76$, $p = .01$. Subjective experience of fear had a trend level significant quadratic relationship, IRR = 1.0003, $z = 1.85$, $p = .06$, such that again at low levels of fear experience (scores lower than 55.06), the relationship between fear experience and antisociality was significant, IRI = 0.96, $z = -1.98$, $p = .05$. Consistent with previous analyses with total ICU scores, the inclusion of both scores on the callous subscale and subjectively experienced fear was a better fitting model for predicting antisociality, AIC = 985.52, BIC = 1007.13, in comparison with the callous subscale only, AIC = 1014.99, BIC = 1029.50. Again, we examined the interaction between callous subscale scores and subjectively experienced fear in the prediction of antisociality. Results revealed no significant interaction between callous subscale scores on the ICU and subjectively experienced fear on antisociality.

DISCUSSION

The current findings provide the first evidence that the intensity of ecologically evoked subjective fear—but not other emotions—significantly predicts antisocial behavior. Our analyses revealed a significant quadratic relationship between subjectively experienced fear and both antisocial behavior and CU traits, such that at low levels of fear experience, decreases in subjectively experienced fear while attending a nationally ranked seasonal haunted attraction, Markoff's Haunted Forest, predicted more serious lifetime antisocial behaviors as well as higher levels of CU traits, a difference that was accounted for primarily by callous subscale scores. Even after controlling for possible shared variance between fear experiences and CU traits, both remained significant predictors of antisociality. Furthermore, the inclusion of fear experience strengthened the overall model predicting antisocial behaviors in comparison to a model with CU traits alone as predictors of antisociality. This pattern of findings was specific to subjectively experienced fear and no other emotional experience or the more general measurement of reduced trait emotionality: the unemotional subscale of the ICU.

These findings illuminate the relevance of fearless traits to the construct of psychopathy through a direct examination of the association between fear experience, CU traits, and a lifetime history of antisocial behaviors in a large community sample. Contrary to theories that fearlessness is unrelated to maladaptive features of psychopathic traits, including aggressive and antisocial behaviors (Miller & Lynam, 2012; Seibert et al., 2011), the current findings suggest an association between lower subjectively experienced fear and more frequent instances of antisocial behaviors. It has been argued that even when associated with antisocial features of psychopathy, fearlessness is relevant to psychopathy only in conjunction with high levels of other affective and interpersonal traits associated with psychopathy, such as callous traits (Lynam & Miller, 2012). However, the association we identified between reduced fear experience and increased antisociality was not explained by associations between fearlessness and other affective and interpersonal traits central to the psychopathy construct, such as CU traits (Kahn, Byrd, & Pardini, 2013; Kimonis et al., 2013; B. A. White et al., 2015). Our analyses revealed a robust relationship between fearlessness and antisociality when both variables were modeled as independent from CU traits and also after controlling for the covariance between CU traits and fearlessness. Moreover, when comparing models predicting antisociality, the addition of subjective fear experience increased the predictive power of the overall model. Together these findings suggest that fearlessness is meaningfully associated with increased antisociality independent from associations with other traits associated with psychopathy. As such, fearlessness at extreme levels may capture a key dimension of the psychopathic personality underlying the emergence of maladaptive behaviors, including antisocial and aggressive behaviors.

These findings suggest that prior findings of fearless traits demonstrating weak associations with antisocial behaviors may reflect insufficiently precise assessments of fearlessness. This possibility is consistent with our finding that, in contrast to our measures of subjectively experienced fearlessness, the unemotional subscale of the ICU demonstrated a nonsignificant association with measurements of antisociality. Other trait-based measures of fearlessness may similarly not be measuring fearlessness specifically and more closely approximate a global reduction in negative emotionality as measured by the unemotional subscale of the ICU (Kimonis et al., 2008, 2013). Of note, consistent with our findings, previous research has also found poor associations between the unemotional subscales and measures of antisocial, aggressive, and delinquent behaviors (Berg et al., 2013; Byrd et al., 2013; Cardinale & Marsh, 2017; Cima, Raine, Meesters, & Popma, 2013; Essau, Sasagawa, & Frick, 2006; Waller et al., 2015), further reinforcing that measuring global reduction of negative emotionality may not capture the key affective traits underlying psychopathy and antisociality. Due to time constraints inherent in the testing environment, the current study did not include lengthier measures of adult psychopathy that have previously been used when assessing the relationship between fearless dominance and maladaptive behavioral traits associated with psychopathy. As a result, the current study cannot directly compare the association between our measure of fear experience and antisociality with the association between other trait-based measures of fearless dominance, such as the fearless-dominance subscale of the Psychopathic Personality Inventory, and antisociality (Lilienfeld, Widows, & P.A.R. Staff, 2005). Future studies should more directly compare the relationships between traditionally used assessments of fearless-dominant traits and antisociality with direct measurements of fear experiences and antisociality.

Another explanation for previous findings of weak associations between fear experience and both antisocial behaviors and CU traits may relate to the nature of the samples typically investigated in studies of fear experience, psychopathy, and antisocial behaviors. It is notable that within our large community sample of adults, the hypothesized relationship between fear experience and both antisociality and CU traits was present only for those who experienced lower than average levels of fear experience, as captured by the quadratic relationships we identified between subjective fear and CU traits and antisociality. This suggests that the nature of the relationship between fearlessness and both antisociality and CU traits may be partially dependent on the range of fearless traits in the sample selected. A sample consisting only of participants reporting average to high levels of fear might not exhibit a significant relationship between fear experience and both antisociality and CU traits. The current study benefited from a large sample size and a wide range of levels of subjective fear experience and CU traits, allowing for an examination of the relationship between these traits and externalizing behaviors across a wide spectrum.

It should also be noted that, as expected, the distribution of antisocial experiences in our sample was strongly skewed such that approximately half of participants reported no instances of physical fights or arrests. As a result, all analyses included Huber-White corrected robust standard errors, and Vuong tests were performed to determine when zero-inflated models should be conducted. The resulting findings can most accurately be generalized to a community population. However, investigation of samples with more consistently high levels of antisocial behaviors (i.e., forensic or clinical samples) should be conducted to further elucidate the relationship between experienced fear and frequent antisocial behaviors. While the study included induction of fear experience, our findings are correlational and thus cannot be used to infer any causal relationships among subjective fear experience, CU traits, and antisocial tendencies as they are measured in the current study. The current study relied on a self-report measure of subjectively experienced fear in Markoff's Haunted Forest. Bolstering confidence in our measure, ratings of subjective fear experiences were closely related to both self-reported measures of sympathetic, but not parasympathetic, activity, and to measures of general fear experience. We were also limited in the number of questions we could ask our participants given the nature of the experimental setting. As such, there remain many additional questions for future research examining individual differences in emotional responses in this fear-inducing environment, including associations with traits such as the ease with which individuals can imagine themselves in fictional situations (a specific domain of dispositional empathy), or clinically relevant symptoms such as depression, which could relate to overall diminished emotional reactivity rather than fear experience specifically. More, our measure of fear experience occurred directly after the fear-inducing event (mean latency = 9.89 min). However, future studies measuring real-time indicators of emotion using, for example, wearable peripheral monitors could add further clarity to our findings.

Finally, the use of Markoff's Haunted Forest as a naturalistic fear induction provided a unique opportunity to study ecologically valid fear experiences. However, with this approach, we lose the precise experimental control possible in laboratory settings. This requires our results to be interpreted in light of the following considerations. First, the walk through the forest was self-guided. Because of this, the 20-minute estimate is based on average consumer behavior, and thus it is possible that various factors such as emotional experience while in the forest could affect the duration of time spent in the forest. Given the current study's focus on subjective experience of fear and the main findings related to reduced fear experience in the forest, it is unlikely that duration of the walk alone could account for our findings. Future research could examine how real-time intensity of emotional experience relates to behaviors such as avoidance while in the forest and thus account for the potential temporal variance in exposure to frightening experiences. In addition to considering more directly the temporal nature of the participants' experience while in the forest, researchers could also assess self-guided emotion regulation strategies as fear is evoked in real time. This would allow for the investigation of individual differences in the use of strategies to downregulate fear. Lastly, we did not conduct research with individuals prior to entering the Haunted Forest and thus cannot assess changes in reported emotional state or personality traits as a function of the fear-inducing experience. But in that our study demonstrates the feasibility of collecting data in a highly fear-evoking setting, it opens the door to various other studies. For example, the causal effects of fear experience could be assessed by comparing responses on measures of constructs believed to be causally influenced by acute fear experience before and after participants enter the forest.

Despite these limitations, the current study provides evidence in support of the role of reduced experience of fear as a potential mechanism for the emergence of antisocial and aggressive behaviors associated with psychopathic traits. Our findings revealed a nonlinear relationship between subjectively experienced fear and both CU traits and antisociality. Within our sample, decreased subjective fear experience was associated with increased antisociality, even after controlling for covariation with CU traits across individuals who experienced below-average levels of fear. These findings have implications for the conceptualization of fearlessness as an emergent property of psychopathic traits that is unrelated to maladaptive features of the psychopathic personality. Instead, our findings support theories that at extreme levels, reduced experience of fear, in conjunction with other interpersonal and affective traits associated with psychopathy (i.e., callousness), may yield heightened risk for antisocial behaviors. Furthermore, our finding that subjective experience of fear specifically, and not the ICU's measure of general poverty of affect or measure of other subjectively experienced emotions, was associated with patterns of antisocial behavior and CU traits suggests that assessments of fear experience specifically and not general trait unemotionality may better capture the core underlying affective deficits associated with psychopathy.

REFERENCES

Berg, J. M., Lilienfeld, S. O., Reddy, S. D., Latzman, R. D., Roose, A., Craighead, L. W., . . . Raison, C. L. (2013). The Inventory of Callous and Unemotional Traits: A construct-validational analysis in an at-risk sample. *Assessment, 20,* 532–544.

Birbaumer, N., Veit, R., Lotze, M., Erb, M., Hermann, C., Grodd, W., & Flor, H. (2005). Deficient fear conditioning in psychopathy: A functional magnetic resonance imaging study. *Archives of General Psychiatry, 62,* 799–805.

Blair, R. J. R. (2005). Applying a cognitive neuroscience perspective to the disorder of psychopathy. *Development and Psychopathology, 17,* 865–891.

Blair, R. J. R. (2013). The neurobiology of psychopathic traits in youths. *Nature Reviews Neuroscience, 14,* 786–799.

Blair, R. J. R., Hwang, S., White, S. F., & Meffert, H. (2016). Emotional learning, psychopathy, and norm development. In S. M. Liao (Ed.), *Moral brains: The neuroscience of morality* (pp. 185–202). New York, NY: Oxford University Press.

Blair, R. J. R., Mitchell, D. G. V., Leonard, A., Budhani, S., Peschardt, K. S., & Newman, C. (2004). Passive avoidance learning in individuals with psychopathy: Modulation by reward but not by punishment. *Personality and Individual Differences, 37,* 1179–1192.

Byrd, A. L., Kahn, R. E., & Pardini, D. A. (2013). A validation of the Inventory of Callous-Unemotional Traits in a community sample of young adult males. *Journal of Psychopathology and Behavioral Assessment, 35*(1). https://doi.org/10.1007/s10862-012-9315-4.

Cardinale, E. M., Breeden, A. L., Robertson, E. L., Lozier, L. M., Vanmeter, J. W., & Marsh, A. A. (2018). Externalizing behavior severity in youths with callous-unemotional traits corresponds to patterns of amygdala activity and connectivity during judgments of causing fear. *Development and Psychopathology, 30*(1), 191-201.

Cardinale, E. M., & Marsh, A. A. (2017). The reliability and validity of the Inventory of Callous-Unemotional Traits: A meta-analytic review. *Assessment, 27,* 57–71.

Cima, M., Raine, A., Meesters, C., & Popma, A. (2013). Validation of the Dutch Reactive Proactive Questionnaire (RPQ): Differential correlates of reactive and proactive aggression from childhood to adulthood. *Aggressive Behavior, 39,* 99–113.

Cleckley, H. (1976). *The mask of sanity* (5th ed.). St. Louis, MO: Mosby.

Decety, J. (2010). The neurodevelopment of empathy in humans. *Developmental Neuroscience, 32,* 257–267.

Drislane, L. E., Brislin, S. J., Kendler, K. S., Andershed, H., Larsson, H., & Patrick, C. J. (2015). A triarchic model analysis of the Youth Psychopathic Traits Inventory. *Journal of Personality Disorders, 29,* 15–41.

Drislane, L. E., Patrick, C. J., & Arsal, G. (2014). Clarifying the content coverage of differing psychopathy inventories through reference to the Triarchic Psychopathy Measure. *Psychological Assessment, 26,* 350–362.

Essau, C. A., Sasagawa, S., & Frick, P. J. (2006). Callous-unemotional traits in a community sample of adolescents. *Assessment, 13,* 454–469.

Fanti, K. A., Panayiotou, G., Lazarou, C., Michael, R., & Georgiou, G. (2016). The better of two evils? Evidence that children exhibiting continuous conduct problems high or low on callous-unemotional traits score on opposite directions on physiological and behavioral measures of fear. *Development and Psychopathology, 28,* 185–198.

Fix, R. L., & Fix, S. T. (2015). Trait psychopathy, emotional intelligence, and criminal thinking: Predicting illegal behavior among college students. *International Journal of Law and Psychiatry, 42–43,* 183–188.

Flor, H., Birbaumer, N., Hermann, C., Ziegler, S., & Patrick, C. (2002). Aversive Pavlovian conditioning in psychopaths: Peripheral and central correlates. *Psychophysiology, 39,* 505–518.

Frick, P. J., & Morris, A. S. (2004). Temperament and developmental pathways to conduct problems. *Journal of Clinical Child and Adolescent Psychology, 33,* 54–68.

Frick, P. J., & Ray, J. V. (2015). Evaluating callous-unemotional traits as a personality construct: Callous-unemotional traits. *Journal of Personality, 83,* 710–722.

Frick, P. J., & White, S. F. (2008). Research review: The importance of callous-unemotional traits for developmental models of aggressive and antisocial behavior. *Journal of Child Psychology and Psychiatry, 49,* 359–375.

Gao, Y., Raine, A., Venables, P. H., Dawson, M. E., & Mednick, S. A. (2009). Association of poor childhood fear conditioning and adult crime. *American Journal of Psychiatry, 167,* 56–60.

Gao, Y., Raine, A., Venables, P. H., Dawson, M. E., & Mednick, S. A. (2010). Reduced electrodermal fear conditioning from ages 3 to 8 years is associated with aggressive behavior at age 8 years. *Journal of Child Psychology and Psychiatry, 51,* 550–558.

Hare, R. D. (1982). Psychopathy and physiological activity during anticipation of an aversive stimulus in a distraction paradigm. *Psychophysiology, 19*, 266–271.

Hare, R. D. (2006). Psychopathy: A clinical and forensic overview. *Psychiatric Clinics of North America, 29*, 709–724.

Hare, R. D., & Neumann, C. S. (2010). The role of antisociality in the psychopathy construct: Comment on Skeem and Cooke (2010). *Psychological Assessment, 22*, 446–454.

Herpertz, S. C., Werth, U., Lukas, G., Qunaibi, M., Schuerkens, A., Kunert, H. J., . . . Sass, H. (2001). Emotion in criminal offenders with psychopathy and borderline personality disorder. *Archives of General Psychiatry, 58*, 737–745.

Joynt, C. R. (2012, October 4). Dead Zone: Behind the scenes at Markoff's Haunted Forest. *Washingtonian*. Retrieved from http://www.washingtonian.com

Kahn, R. E., Byrd, A. L., & Pardini, D. A. (2013). Callous-unemotional traits robustly predict future criminal offending in young men. *Law and Human Behavior, 37*, 87–97.

Kimonis, E. R., Branch, J., Hagman, B., Graham, N., & Miller, C. (2013). The psychometric properties of the Inventory of Callous-Unemotional Traits in an undergraduate sample. *Psychological Assessment, 25*, 84–93.

Kimonis, E. R., Fanti, K. A., Goulter, N., & Hall, J. (2017). Affective startle potentiation differentiates primary and secondary variants of juvenile psychopathy. *Development and Psychopathology, 29*, 1149–1160.

Kimonis, E. R., Frick, P. J., Skeem, J. L., Marsee, M. A., Cruise, K., Munoz, L. C., . . . Morris, A. S. (2008). Assessing callous-unemotional traits in adolescent offenders: Validation of the Inventory of Callous-Unemotional Traits. *International Journal of Law and Psychiatry, 31*, 241–252.

Kochanska, G., Gross, J. N., Lin, M. H., & Nichols, K. E. (2002). Guilt in young children: Development, determinants, and relations with a broader system of standards. *Child Development, 73*, 461–482.

Leistico, A. M. R., Salekin, R. T., DeCoster, J., & Rogers, R. (2008). A large-scale meta-analysis relating the Hare measures of psychopathy to antisocial conduct. *Law and Human Behavior, 32*, 28–45.

Levenson, M. R., Kiehl, K. A., & Fitzpatrick, C. M. (1995). Assessing psychopathic attributes in a noninstitutionalized population. *Journal of Personality and Social Psychology, 68*, 151–158.

Levenston, G. K., Patrick, C. J., Bradley, M. M., & Lang, P. J. (2000). The psychopath as observer: Emotion and attention in picture processing. *Journal of Abnormal Psychology, 109*, 373–385.

Lilienfeld, S. O., & Andrews, B. P. (1996). Development and preliminary validation of a self-report measure of psychopathic personality traits in noncriminal population. *Journal of Personality Assessment, 66*, 488–524.

Lilienfeld, S. O., Patrick, C. J., Benning, S. D., Berg, J., Sellbom, M., & Edens, J. F. (2012). The role of fearless dominance in psychopathy: Confusions, controversies, and clarifications. *Personality Disorders, 3*, 327–340.

Lilienfeld, S. O., Smith, S. F., Sauvigné, K. C., Patrick, C. J., Drislane, L. E., Latzman, R. D., & Krueger, R. F. (2016). Is boldness relevant to psychopathic personality? Meta-analytic relations with non-Psychopathy Checklist-based measures of psychopathy. *Psychological Assessment, 28*, 1172–1185.

Lilienfeld, S. O., Widows, M. R., & P.A.R. Staff. (2005). Psychopathic Personality Inventory TM-Revised. *Social Influence (SOI), 61*(65), 97.

Long, J. S., & Freese, J. (2006). *Regression models for categorical dependent variables using Stata* (2nd ed.). College Station, TX: Stata Press.

Lorber, M. F. (2004). Psychophysiology of aggression, psychopathy, and conduct problems: A meta-analysis. *Psychological Bulletin, 130*, 531–552.

Lykken, D. T. (1957). A study of anxiety in the sociopathic personality. *Journal of Abnormal Psychology, 55*(1), 6–10.

Lykken, D. T. (2013). *The antisocial personalities*. New York, NY: Psychology Press.

Lynam, D. R., & Miller, J. D. (2012). Fearless dominance and psychopathy: A response to Lilienfeld et al. *Personality Disorders, 3*, 341–353.

Marcus, D. K., Fulton, J. J., & Edens, J. F. (2013). The two-factor model of psychopathic personality: Evidence from the Psychopathic Personality Inventory. *Personality Disorders, 4*, 67–76.

Marsh, A. A. (2018). The neuroscience of empathy. *Current Opinion in Behavioral Sciences, 19*, 110–115. https://doi.org/10.1016/j.cobeha.2017.12.016

Marsh, A. A., & Cardinale, E. M. (2012). Psychopathy and fear: Specific impairments in judging behaviors that frighten others. *Emotion, 12*, 892–898.

Marsh, A. A., & Cardinale, E. M. (2014). When psychopathy impairs moral judgments: Neural responses during judgments about causing fear. *Social Cognitive and Affective Neuroscience, 9*, 3–11.

Marsh, A. A., Finger, E. C., Schechter, J. C., Jurkowitz, I. T., Reid, M. E., & Blair, R. J. (2011). Adolescents with psychopathic traits report reductions in physiological responses to fear. *Journal of Child Psychology and Psychiatry, 52*, 834–841.

Miller, J. D., & Lynam, D. R. (2012). An examination of the Psychopathic Personality Inventory's nomological network: A meta-analytic review. *Personality Disorders, 3*, 305–326.

Ortiz, J., & Raine, A. (2004). Heart rate level and antisocial behavior in children and adolescents: A meta-analysis. *Journal of the American Academy of Child & Adolescent Psychiatry, 43*, 154–162.

Patrick, C. J., Venables, N. C., & Drislane, L. E. (2013). The role of fearless dominance in differentiating psychopathy from antisocial personality disorder: Comment on Marcus, Fulton, and Edens. *Personality Disorders, 4*, 80–82.

Raine, A. (1996). Autonomic nervous system factors underlying disinhibited, antisocial, and violent behavior. Biosocial perspectives and treatment implications. *Annals of the New York Academy of Sciences, 794*, 46–59.

Raine, A. (2002). Annotation: The role of prefrontal deficits, low autonomic arousal, and early health factors in the development of antisocial and aggressive behavior in children. *Journal of Child Psychology and Psychiatry, 43*(4), 417-434.

Raine, A., Dodge, K., Loeber, R., Gatzke-Kopp, L., Lynam, D., Reynolds, C., . . . Liu, J. (2006). The Reactive-Proactive Aggression Questionnaire: Differential correlates of reactive and proactive aggression in adolescent boys. *Aggressive Behavior, 32*, 159–171.

Rothemund, Y., Ziegler, S., Hermann, C., Gruesser, S. M., Foell, J., Patrick, C. J., & Flor, H. (2012). Fear conditioning in psychopaths: Event-related potentials and peripheral measures. *Biological Psychology, 90*, 50–59.

Schenk, A. M., Ragatz, L. L., & Fremouw, W. J. (2012). Vicious dogs part 2: Criminal thinking, callousness, and personality styles of their owners. *Journal of Forensic Science, 57*, 152–159.

Scherer, K. R., & Wallbott, H. G. (1994). Evidence for universality and cultural variation of differential emotion response patterning. *Journal of Personality and Social Psychology, 66*, 310–328.

Seibert, L. A., Miller, J. D., Few, L. R., Zeichner, A., & Lynam, D. R. (2011). An examination of the structure of self-report psychopathy measures and their relations with general traits and externalizing behaviors. *Personality Disorders, 2*, 193–208.

Stoeber, J. (2015). How other-oriented perfectionism differs from self-oriented and socially prescribed perfectionism: Further findings. *Journal of Psychopathology and Behavorial Assessment, 37*, 611–623.

Thomson, N. D., Aboutanos, M., Kiehl, K. A., Neumann, C., Galusha, C., & Fanti, K. A. (2018). Physiological reactivity in response to a fear-induced virtual reality experience: Associations with psychopathic traits. *Psychophysiology, 56*(1), e13276.

Waller, R., Shaw, D. S., & Hyde, L. W. (2017). Observed fearlessness and positive parenting interact to predict childhood callous-unemotional behaviors among low-income boys. *Journal of Child Psychology and Psychiatry, 58*, 282–291. https://doi.org/10.1111/jcpp.12666

Waller, R., Wright, A. G., Shaw, D. S., Gardner, F., Dishion, T. J., Wilson, M. N., & Hyde, L. W. (2015). Factor structure and construct validity of the Parent-Reported Inventory of Callous-Unemotional Traits among high-risk 9-year-olds. *Assessment, 22*, 561–580.

White, A. C., & Miller, C. J. (2014). Delinquency in emerging adult females: The importance of callous-unemotionality and impulsivity. *Deviant Behavior, 36*, 245–258.

White, B. A., Gordon, H., & Guerra, R. C. (2015). Callous-unemotional traits and empathy in proactive and reactive relational aggression in young women. *Personality and Individual Differences, 75*, 185–189.

White, S. F., Briggs-Gowan, M. J., Voss, J. L., Petitclerc, A., McCarthy, K., Blair, R. J. R., & Wakschlag, L. S. (2016). Can the fear recognition deficits associated with callous-unemotional traits be identified in early childhood? *Journal of Clinical and Experimental Neuropsychology, 38*, 672–684.

Beliefs about Emotion Shift Dynamically Alongside Momentary Affect

Jennifer C. Veilleux, PhD, Elise A. Warner, MSW,
Danielle E. Baker, MA, and Kaitlyn D. Chamberlain, MA

> This study examined if beliefs about emotion change across emotional contexts in daily life, and it investigated whether people with prominent features of borderline personality pathology experience greater shifts in emotion beliefs during emotional states. Undergraduate participants with (n = 49) and without borderline features (n = 50) completed a 1-week ecological momentary assessment study where they provided ratings of affect, nine different beliefs about emotion, and indicators of momentary self-efficacy. Results support the notion of beliefs as relatively schematic. However, most of the beliefs about emotion shifted with either positive or negative affect, and they predicted momentary self-efficacy for tolerating distress and exerting willpower. Those with borderline features experienced greater instability of beliefs, and borderline features moderated the relationships between affect and many beliefs. Results confirm that there are implications for emotion beliefs for people who struggle with emotion regulation and impulsivity (i.e., people with features of borderline personality).
>
> *Keywords:* affect, emotion beliefs, emotion schemas, borderline personality, ecological momentary assessment

People have beliefs about emotions—both their own emotions and how emotions work in general—and these beliefs matter for understanding the ways people engage with and try to regulate their affective experience (Ford & Gross, 2018, 2019). For example, compared to believing that emotions are fixed (i.e., out of one's control), believing that emotions are controllable (i.e., can be altered with effort) tends to be associated with higher levels of well-being (De Castella et al., 2013; Tamir, John, Srivastava, & Gross, 2007), more active emotion regulation efforts (De Castella et al., 2013; Gutentag, Halperin, Porat, Bigman, & Tamir, 2016; Kneeland, Nolen-Hoeksema, Dovidio, & Gruber, 2016), and fewer symptoms of psychopathology (Kneeland, Dovidio, Joormann, & Clark, 2016). Other beliefs, which are often described as emotional schemas (Leahy, 2002, 2015, 2016), include beliefs that emotions

From University of Arkansas, Fayetteville, Arkansas.

Address correspondence to Jennifer C. Veilleux, PhD, Associate Professor, Department of Psychological Science, University of Arkansas, 216 Memorial Hall, Fayetteville, AR 72703. E-mail: jcveille@uark.edu

Originally published in the *Journal of Personality Disorders*, Volume 35, Supplement A. ©2021 The Guilford Press.

last "forever," that emotions should be simple and not complex, and that emotions should not be expressed to others (Veilleux, Chamberlain, Baker, & Warner, 2019). In general, more extreme and harsh beliefs about emotion (i.e., beliefs that emotions will last forever, that emotional expression is dangerous, that your own emotions are different from other peoples') are thought to be maladaptive, because these beliefs are associated with a host of problematic outcomes, including engagement in impulsive behaviors (Manser, Cooper, & Trefusis, 2012), difficulties effectively regulating emotions (Veilleux, Pollert, et al., 2019; Veilleux, Salomaa, Shaver, Zielinski, & Pollert, 2015) and increases in psychopathology (see Edwards & Wupperman, 2019, and Ford & Gross, 2018, for reviews). Thus, beliefs about emotion have important implications for emotional well-being (Ford & Gross, 2019).

Many questions remain about the nature and implications of emotion beliefs (Edwards & Wupperman, 2019; Ford & Gross, 2018). One central question is whether beliefs about emotions are stable across time and context. Typically, beliefs have been considered as an individual difference, where one person ("Petra") has strong beliefs that emotions are "fixed" and another person ("Kim") has strong beliefs that emotions are malleable (Tamir et al., 2007). People may vary in their level of belief across different belief dimensions. For example, although Petra would be identified as holding a more maladaptive malleability belief, Petra also believes that emotions are meant to be shared with others (a generally adaptive perspective; Kennedy-Moore & Watson, 2001). Essentially, although people may differ along each belief dimension, the general notion is that a person *has* a belief. This is consistent with thinking of beliefs as "schematic"—core, unchanging perspectives that a person holds about the world (Cervone, 2004).

Yet it is also possible that beliefs about emotion actually change over time and across contexts, particularly negative emotional contexts. Most people experience mild positive affect as their "typical" emotional state (Yik, Russell, & Barrett, 1999). If emotion beliefs are schematic individual differences, we would expect people to report similar beliefs in this "typical" emotional state as when they are experiencing a strong emotion. However, it seems likely that at least *some* people may experience changes in beliefs when in a strong emotional state. Consider Raul, who at a typical moment would report strong beliefs that people can behave effectively even when experiencing a strong emotion. When Raul gets mad or frustrated with himself, however, he gives up on his tasks easily. If we were to assess his belief when he is frustrated, he might be more likely to endorse the belief that he cannot act effectively because of his emotional state. Understanding *if* beliefs change across contexts, *for whom* beliefs change, *which* beliefs change across *which contexts*, and the *implications* of momentary beliefs could provide valuable information for understanding how beliefs contribute to emotional experience and emotion regulation efforts.

Can beliefs change over time? We think yes. When asked, "Do your beliefs change when you experience a strong emotion?" about two thirds of people answer yes (Veilleux, Pollert, et al., 2019). This type of simple self-report data is not actual evidence demonstrating fluctuations in beliefs, but it does suggest that most people *think* their beliefs change during emotional states. The ideal way to assess actual belief changeability is by ecological momentary assessment (EMA), where people repeatedly report on emotions and beliefs about emotion across time while living their daily lives (Santangelo, Bohus, & Ebner-Priemer, 2014; Shiffman, Stone, & Hufford, 2008). Recent work using EMA has demonstrated that attributes long investigated as individual differences, such as impulsivity (Tomko et al., 2014), distress tolerance (Veilleux et al., 2018), and even personality traits (Howell, Ksendzova, Nestingen, Yerahian, & Iyer, 2017; Wilson, Thompson, & Vazire, 2017) demonstrate variability across time and contexts. The time is thus ripe for examination of the dynamics of emotion beliefs.

Who is likely to experience greater belief changeability during emotional situations? Our sense is that people who become overly absorbed by and are highly reactive to their emotions and who experience rapid shifts in cognition during emotional events are probably also prone to their beliefs changing in strong emotional states. This description is consistent with symptoms of borderline personality disorder (BPD), which is characterized by elevated frequency, intensity, and duration of negative emotions (Chu, Victor, & Klonsky, 2016), as well as greater affective instability (Santangelo et al., 2014) and more negative self-focused thoughts (Baer, Peters, Eisenlohr-Moul, Geiger, & Sauer, 2012). In addition, more maladaptive beliefs about emotion (i.e., stronger beliefs that emotions last forever, beliefs that emotions should be hidden from others, beliefs that emotions cannot be changed, and beliefs that other people do not feel the same emotions) are associated with increased symptoms of BPD (Veilleux, Chamberlain, et al., 2019; Veilleux, Pollert, et al., 2019). These findings all suggest that heightened emotional intensity and maladaptive beliefs likely co-occur for people with greater BPD symptoms. Research also suggests that people with BPD demonstrate greater variability in thoughts about themselves (i.e., self-worth) and others compared to healthy controls (Kanske et al., 2016; Tolpin, Gunthert, Cohen, & O'Neill, 2004; Zeigler-Hill & Abraham, 2006). Finally, experimental evidence suggests that thought processes and problem-solving abilities shift during negative affect for people with BPD (Dixon-Gordon, Chapman, Lovasz, & Walters, 2011). Taken together, these findings lend support for considering people with elevated BPD symptoms as a potential target group who may experience belief changeability.

Which beliefs will change across which contexts? We have already stated that our prediction is that beliefs will become stronger and likely more maladaptive during stronger negative emotional states. Yet the question remains as to *which* beliefs will fluctuate with emotion. Controllability is a likely candidate, considering that controllability beliefs have been successfully manipulated and shown to cause changes in emotion regulation strategies (Kneeland, Nolen-Hoeksema, et al., 2016). However, considering the wide range of beliefs people *can* hold about emotion, perhaps it makes more sense to assess a variety of emotion beliefs to examine which beliefs do and which do not change across contexts. A new tool (Individual Beliefs About Emotion; Veilleux, Chamberlain, et al., 2019), derived from clinical material about emotion "myths" (Leahy, Tirch, & Napolitano, 2011; Linehan, 2015; Spradlin, 2003), assesses nine different beliefs about emotion with one item each. This is ideal for use in EMA, where assessments should be brief to minimize burden for participants repeatedly completing measures during daily life (Shiffman et al., 2008; Trull & Ebner-Priemer, 2013). The nine beliefs include the belief that emotions come from "out of the blue" (beliefs about the cause of emotions), that negative emotions are bad and destructive (judgment beliefs), that emotions should be simple (complexity), that emotions should not be shared with others (expression), that logic is preferable to emotion (preference), that emotions control behavior, that emotions cannot be changed (malleability), that one's own emotions are different from other people's emotions (uniqueness), and that emotions "last forever" (longevity). Prior work has shown that these beliefs predict relevant emotional outcomes such that more maladaptive beliefs tend to be associated with greater symptoms of psychological distress and borderline personality symptoms (Veilleux, Chamberlain, et al., 2019; Veilleux, Pollert, et al., 2019), as well as emotion dysregulation, lower emotional expressivity, lower mindfulness, and lower emotional intelligence (Veilleux, Pollert, et al., 2019). Examining a variety of beliefs simultaneously could allow for a nuanced examination of how different beliefs about emotion shift across time and situation.

Finally, what are the implications of emotion beliefs for momentary self-regulation decisions? A person who believes that negative emotions are bad and/or that emotions cannot be changed is less likely to pursue active emotion regulation and more likely to try to avoid or escape his or her feelings (De Castella, Platow, Tamir, & Gross, 2018; Ford & Gross, 2018, 2019; Kneeland, Nolen-Hoeksema, et al., 2016). Emotion beliefs may also be related to a sense of self-efficacy for managing emotional situations, including momentary perceptions of the ability to tolerate distress (Veilleux et al., 2018), as well as people's momentary sense of whether they are capable of exerting willpower to achieve their goals (Veilleux, Skinner, Baker, & Chamberlain, 2019). Although both beliefs about emotion and distress tolerance have been described as conveying negative attitudes about emotion (Yoon, Dang, Mertz, & Rottenberg, 2018), they are empirically distinct at least in terms of predicting depression (Yoon et al., 2018). Moreover, whereas beliefs about emotion assess beliefs about how emotions operate either in general (Tamir et al., 2007; Veilleux et al., 2015) or specific to the person (De Castella et al., 2013), they do not address a person's own sense of agency in responding to those emotions, whether in terms of sitting with the emotions (i.e., distress tolerance) or exerting self-control toward goals (i.e., willpower). Considering that people who feel self-efficacious are more likely to engage in the behavior they feel capable of accomplishing (Bandura, 2001; Cervone, 2000), momentary distress tolerance and momentary willpower may be useful self-efficacy constructs to assess in relation to emotion beliefs. Distress tolerance and difficulties engaging in goal-directed behavior are two of the central difficulties for people with BPD (Selby & Joiner, 2009), as well as comorbid conditions such as depression (Kotov et al., 2017). Thus the relationship between these indicators of self-regulatory self-efficacy and emotion beliefs may be particularly prominent for those with heightened BPD features.

In the current study, our goals were to determine *if* beliefs change across contexts, evaluate *which* beliefs change across contexts, provide an initial examination of *for whom* beliefs change *in which emotional contexts*, and examine the *implications* of emotion beliefs on momentary self-efficacy to tolerate distress and engage in self-control. We predicted that beliefs would change over time to a greater degree for people with significant features of borderline personality compared to those without borderline features. We thought it likely that some of the beliefs would change more than others, but we did not have specific a priori predictions as to which beliefs would be more variable. We also predicted that momentary beliefs about emotion would vary based on emotional context, where we predicted that higher negative and lower positive affect would be associated with stronger maladaptive beliefs, and that the relationships between beliefs and affect—particularly negative affect—would be stronger for people with borderline features. Finally, to understand some of the implications for emotion beliefs for self-efficacy, we examined the set of nine emotion beliefs predicting both momentary distress intolerance and momentary willpower. Considering that beliefs about malleability have been linked to avoidance-based emotion regulation (De Castella et al., 2018; Kneeland, Nolen-Hoeksema, et al., 2016) and beliefs about emotion longevity (i.e., that emotions will last "forever") seem to be particularly prominent for BPD (Veilleux, Chamberlain, et al., 2019), we predicted that malleability and longevity beliefs would predict momentary distress intolerance particularly for people with borderline features. We also expected that beliefs about behavior control would be uniquely predictive of willpower.

METHODS

Recruitment

Participants were recruited from an undergraduate psychology subject pool using a prescreening measure that included the Personality Assessment Inventory-Borderline Features Scale (PAI-BOR; Morey, 1991). The scale has 24 items given on a 4-point scale with ratings of *False*, *Slightly True*, *Moderately True*, and *Very True*. The scale has been used previously to detect individuals with significant features of borderline personality disorder (Trull, 1995; Trull, Useda, Conforti, & Doan, 1997), such that individuals with a *T* score of 70 or greater experience significant BPD features indicative of high emotional intensity and emotional reactivity, difficulties with self-control and emotion regulation, and significant interpersonal distress. We recruited people with *T* scores of 70 or greater (raw scores 38 or higher) as the BPD features group and people with scores below 60 (raw scores 27 or below) for the comparison group. We intentionally call the comparison group the non-BPD group rather than assuming these are "healthy controls" because we did not assess or exclude people based on other forms of psychopathology (e.g., depression, anxiety). In total, we screened 2,178 individuals from the subject pool, where 16.6% had *T* scores of 70 or above and 58.5% had *T* scores below 60. Although we recognize that recruiting based on extreme groups is perhaps less ideal than recruiting the entire range of scores and oversampling for high scores (Fisher, Guha, Heller, & Miller, 2020), our goals here were to examine groups as a proxy for diagnosis, and the selected sampling strategy included many people in the midrange of scores as recommended when using extreme groups analysis (Fisher et al., 2020).

Once screened, participants were invited to sign up for the study, where we opened up slots for 50% with BPD features and the other 50% as the comparison group. Because the screening information also included participants' self-reported gender, we were also able to match the groups based on gender. In total, 105 participants completed the initial visit. Of these, one did not actually have a smartphone and thus was ineligible for the EMA study, and two other participants were accidentally invited but did not actually meet PAI-BOR criteria. In total, 102 participants (BPD features $n = 50$, Non-BPD $n = 52$) completed the 1-week EMA study (72.3% women, mean age 19.30 [$SD = 2.12$], 75.5% White). This sample size was consistent with our a priori sample size goals, which were to obtain 50 people per recruitment group.[1]

Procedure

Participants who met inclusion criteria were invited to the lab for an initial orientation session where they first completed individual difference measures using Qualtrics on a desktop computer. Participants were then guided to chart their emotional episodes as an assessment of emotion dynamics (Kuppens, Oravecz, & Tuerlinckx, 2010). They were first oriented to the chart itself, which has time on the X-axis and emotion on the Y-axis (from 0 to 100). We focused on the emotions of "distress" and "happiness" to broadly encompass negative and positive affect, but using more lay terminology. Participants were told the purpose of the chart was to examine how their emotions often rise and fall around emotional events. They were guided to describe a distressing event and to chart the "wave" of emotion they experienced in response to that distress event, including their starting distress level, the quickness of response, peak response, and time to return to baseline (Kuppens & Verduyn, 2015). They did a similar chart for an experience of happiness. Participants were then asked to identify their usual "distress homebase" and "happiness homebase" where most people tend to have a fairly low "homebase" level of distress (e.g., 10 on a 100-point scale) and a moderate "homebase" level of happiness (e.g., 40 on a 100-point scale). Experimenters recorded the stated distress and happiness "homebases" for each person.

Participants were then introduced to LifeData, the EMA phone application that was used for data collection. LifeData is free for participants and is available on both iPhone and Android operating systems. An orientation session familiarized participants with what to expect in the upcoming week when they were prompted, and a trained research assistant answered any questions participants had about the experiment. Specifically, participants were encouraged to identify their current emotion and determine whether they felt consistent with their homebase (e.g., within 10–20 points of their homebase) or different (either higher or lower) than their homebase. Participants were

---

1. Although a small sample size for traditional between-subject analyses, we anticipated that this sample size would be sufficient for EMA analyses. Power for EMA is complex because of the within-subject and between-subject components in intensive longitudinal data, where Monte Carlo simulations are recommended for power analysis (Bolger & Laurenceau, 2013). We anticipated that 30–50 data points per person would result in more than 3,000 data points, which should be sufficient to conduct this initial evaluation of belief dynamics such that Monte Carlo simulations could be used to establish power for future studies.

also instructed to initiate a prompt when experiencing an emotion different from either their happiness or distress homebase.

After completing the orientation session, the participant was allowed to leave the lab and the week of EMA began. Participants were notified randomly seven times a day for 7 days during the hours of 9:30 a.m. to 9:30 p.m., and they were prompted once daily at 9:35 p.m. to complete nightly entries. At this nightly entry, participants were asked how many emotions they experienced that they neglected to log into the app and to describe why they missed logging. Finally, they were asked if they had any difficulty responding to the prompts that day and, if so, to explain the problems experienced in the format of a free-text response. They also reported on daily stressors experienced (Brantley, Waggoner, Jones, & Rappaport, 1987) and daily participation in creative activities; these nightly entries were not examined in the current set of analyses.

After completing the week-long EMA session, participants came in for a final half-hour debriefing session where they completed a semistructured interview in which they were guided to reflect on what they learned about themselves monitoring their emotions and beliefs over the course of a week. Compensation was in the form of research credits toward a course requirement, with full credit given for completing 80% of random responses, and titrated credit for lower response rates.

Measures

Note that only the measures pertinent to the current analyses are reported here, but the full list of measures given at baseline and by EMA are available at https://osf.io/d7r38/?view_only=82f947abc2f14acda64d4c099a3d6745.

Individual Beliefs About Emotion (IBAE)

The IBAE (Veilleux, Chamberlain, et al., 2019) assesses nine different beliefs about emotion with a single item each. Beliefs are rated from 1 to 5, with different anchors given for each belief. Note that for each measure, anchors are not provided for the middle scores (2–4). All beliefs, questions, and anchors are listed in Table 1. All items were eventually scored such that the less adaptive belief represents the high end to facilitate interpretation. The beliefs measured by the IBAE overlap significantly, with cognitive concepts of emotions assessed as emotional schemas (Leahy, 2002), and greater adherence to maladaptive beliefs predicts symptoms of psychopathology as well as symptoms of borderline personality (Veilleux, Chamberlain, et al., 2019).

EMA Measures

Random Prompts. At each prompt, participants were asked the same set of questions. First, they were asked to rate their current emotion beliefs on the IBAE (see Measures section above). After rating beliefs, participants were asked to report on how they felt on 12 emotional adjectives, 6 positive (joyful, calm, relaxed, excited, proud, happy) and 6 negative (sad, angry, anxious,

TABLE 1. Individual Beliefs About Emotion Items and Anchors

	Construct	Question	Adaptive Anchor	Less Adaptive Anchor
1.	Cause[a]	Where do emotions come from?	Emotions happen because of clear, identifiable causes.	Emotions come from out of the blue, for no reason.
2.	Judgment	What is your attitude toward negative emotions?	Negative feelings are helpful and useful; I welcome my negative feelings.	Negative feelings are bad and destructive; I would prefer to never feel bad.
3.	Complexity	Should emotions be simple or complex?	I can feel a variety of conflicting emotions at once.	I should only feel one thing at a time.
4.	Expression	Should emotions be shared with others?	Emotions must be "let out" and expressed to the world.	Emotions should be kept inside the self; no one wants to deal with other people's emotions.
5.	Preference	Which do you prefer, thought or feeling?	Feeling is preferable to effortful thought.	Logic is preferable to emotion.
6.	Behavior Control[a]	Do emotions control behavior?	It is possible, maybe even easy, to act differently than how I feel inside.	It is extremely hard, maybe impossible, to act differently than what my emotions tell me to do.
7.	Malleability[a]	Can emotions be changed?	Everyone can learn to control their emotions.	Emotions have to "run their course"; they are hard to change or alter.
8.	Uniqueness	Are your emotions different from other peoples?	My emotions are similar to everyone else's.	No one seems to experience emotions the way I do.
9.	Longevity[a]	How long do negative feelings last?	Negative feelings are difficult but don't last very long.	Negative feelings seem to last forever.

[a]Items were presented to participants with the less adaptive anchor on the low side (1); all other items keyed with the less adaptive anchor on the high side (5).

ashamed, jealous, guilty). They rated each adjective on a visual analogue scale from 0 (*Not at all*) to 100 (*Extremely*). Participants were then asked three questions to assess momentary distress tolerance (Veilleux et al., 2018) such as "I want to stop what I'm doing right now so I can feel better" and "Right now, my emotions are getting in my way" on a 7-point Likert scale from 1 (*Strongly disagree*) and 7 (*Strongly agree*). It is important to note that these items assess perceptions of momentary abilities and do not assess actual efforts to tolerate or avoid emotions. Participants were then asked two questions about state willpower, including "How much willpower do you have right now?" and "If I had to do a task right now that required significant self-control, I would be successful at that task" with response options ranging from 0 (*Zero*) to 6 (*Extremely*). (Veilleux, Skinner, et al., 2019).

Participants also completed other measures that are not included in the current analyses, including location and activity when they received the prompt, whether they were experiencing subjectively more distress or happiness than their homebase feeling, and their goals for their emotions. All items presented to participants are listed in the codebook linked above.

Emotion Prompts. Participants were asked to initiate a prompt when they experienced a strong emotion. This kind of "user-initiated session" is common in substance use (e.g., smoking) and eating research (Goldschmidt et al., 2012; Shiffman et al., 2002). In this study, participants were trained to recognize deviations from their baseline during the initial laboratory session (see below). They were first asked to confirm that they were experiencing a strong emotion (yes or no), and then they saw the same questions as in the random prompts.

Data Analytic Strategy

All data for both person-level and EMA analyses are available at https://osf.io/d7r38/?view_only=82f947abc2f14acda64d4c099a3d6745. We first examined response rates to the study and excluded participants with response rates under 30%, which suggested lack of compliance with the EMA protocol. After this, we excluded any EMA "session" (i.e., response to momentary prompt) that was not completed within 10 minutes of receiving the prompt or where most of the data were missing from that session. We then calculated session-level scores for positive affect (average scores on joyful, calm, relaxed, excited, proud, and happy), negative affect (average scores on sad, angry, anxious, ashamed, jealous, guilty), momentary distress intolerance (average scores on the three momentary distress tolerance items), and momentary willpower (average of two momentary willpower items). We then examined the frequency of emotion logs, or how often participants chose to report an emotion. Because the frequency of these reports was very low (121 total emotions logged across all participants, and only 90 of these were "confirmed" to be strong emotions according to their own self-reports), we ultimately combined the emotion logged sessions into an overall data set along with the random prompt sessions. We used chi-square and independent samples t tests to compare differences between the non-BPD group and the BPD features group on demographic variables, reports of homebase levels of distress and happiness, and aggregated momentary variables calculated per person by averaging individuals' momentary responses across the EMA week.

Prior to analyses, the beliefs were scored so that higher scores always reflected more maladaptive outcomes (i.e., Cause, Control Behavior, Malleability, and Longevity were reverse scored). Notably, because the beliefs were assessed with individual items, we could not use traditional psychometric indices (e.g., Cronbach's alpha) to evaluate consistency of measurement. Instead, to evaluate stability or consistency of beliefs, we compared baseline beliefs assessed at the initial lab session and aggregated momentary beliefs over the EMA period by correlation and paired samples t tests. We also looked at both within- and between-person correlations of the momentary belief data using the 'psych' package in R.

We initially assessed variability in the beliefs in two ways. First, we calculated intraclass correlation coefficients (ICCs) to examine the total variance due to mean differences between people—higher scores here reflect greater between-person variability, whereas lower values represent greater within-person variability. Typical daily diary or experience sampling studies have values of .20 to .40 (Bolger & Laurenceau, 2013), reflective of variability over time (i.e., greater within-person than between-person variability). The estimates presented are point estimates with a 95% confidence interval around the point estimate. To examine differences in ICC across groups, we calculated the ICC and confidence intervals for each group and whether the confidence intervals for each group overlapped or not; nonoverlapping confidence intervals suggest differences in ICC across groups. Second, we calculated mean-squared successive difference (MSSD) scores for each belief, which assesses instability (i.e., variability but accounting for time). The MSSD is considered a better index of variation than within-person standard deviation because the MSSD accounts for temporal dependence as well as both the level (i.e., amplitude) and the frequency of assessment (Ebner-Priemer, Eid, Kleindienst, Stabenow, & Trull, 2009; Miller, Vachon, & Lynam, 2009). MSSD is especially useful for within-day successive change, so we calculated an MSSD for each day (the squared successive difference between values in a given day for each person) and then calculated an overall MSSD to represent the average variability across the week. Calculation of MSSD scores allowed us to use independent samples t tests to determine if people in the BPD features group had greater variability in beliefs compared to people in the non-BPD group.

The majority of the analyses were conducted using multilevel modeling to account for the nested data structure, where affect and beliefs were assessed at the momentary level (Level 1), nested within individuals (Level 2). All analyses were conducted in R using package 'lme4,' which uses restricted maximum likelihood to estimate linear mixed effects. The first set of analyses examined the influence of momentary positive and negative affect on beliefs by entering both positive and negative affect simultaneously to predict each belief, along with BPD group (BPD features coded as 1 vs. non-BPD features coded as 0) and the interactions of BPD group with affect to examine whether the relationships between affect and momentary emotion beliefs differed for people with and without borderline features. In these models, Level 1 predictors (positive and negative affect) were person-mean centered (Bolger & Laurenceau, 2013). All fixed effects are presented in the Results tables, simple slopes for significant interactions are presented in the text, and figures are provided depicting significant interactions. Of note, random intercepts were included in all models but random slopes were not, because inclusion of random slopes resulted in nonconvergence, even after testing for singularity, examining gradient calculations, increasing the number of iterations used in the model, and using multiple optimizers.

Finally, to examine the implications of beliefs about emotion for momentary self-efficacy, we conducted two multilevel models predicting momentary distress intolerance and momentary willpower, which each included BPD group, the set of nine beliefs, interactions between BPD group and each belief, and negative affect. Negative affect was included as a control, because prior work found that momentary distress intolerance is higher (Veilleux et al., 2018) and subjective momentary willpower is lower (Veilleux, Skinner, et al., 2019) alongside higher negative affect. All continuous predictors (negative affect, beliefs) were person-mean-centered prior to analyses.

RESULTS

Although 102 eligible participants completed the study, three were excluded for response rates of less than 30%, leaving a final sample size of 99 (BPD features n = 50, Non-BPD n = 49). Demographic information overall and data by recruitment group are presented in Table 2. There were no significant differences in age, percentage female, or percentage minority between the non-BPD and BPD features groups. On average, participants responded to 75.34% of the random prompts (SD = 16.17), with a higher response rate from the non-BPD group compared to the BPD group (see Table 1). In total, 3,975 sessions were logged, with the vast majority of these (97.1%) from random prompts, with the rest from participant-initiated sessions. Overall, 291 of all of the sessions (7.32%) represented "emotion" sessions, where participants indicated they were currently experiencing or had just experienced a strong emotion. Of these "emotion" sessions, more of them (55.6%) were reported by people in the BPD features group compared to the non-BPD group (44.3%), χ^2 = 6.68, p = 01.

TABLE 2. Demographics, Average Responses, and Individual Differences by Recruitment Group

	Total (n = 99)	Non-BPD Group (n = 49) M [SD]	BPD Features Group (n = 50) M [SD]	t (or χ^2)	p
Age	19.32 (2.15)	19.73 (2.85)	18.92 (1.01)	1.89	.06
% Women	71.4	68.8	74.0	χ^2 = .33	.56
% Minority	24.2	26.5	22.0	χ^2 = .27	.60
PAI-BOR	**31.74 (13.83)**	**19.31 (6.48)**	**43.94 (5.92)**	**19.76**	**< .001**
Daily RR	**75.34 (16.16)**	**79.74 (12.80)**	**71.02 (17.99)**	**2.77**	**.01**
Reported "Homebase" Distress	**20.65 (12.98)**	**14.61 (8.09)**	**26.56 (14.16)**	**5.14**	**< .001**
Reported "Homebase" Happiness	41.29 (17.08)	43.27 (17.83)	39.36 (16.24)	1.14	.26
Avg. NA	**19.49 (12.80)**	**13.61 (8.97)**	**25.26 (13.43)**	**5.61**	**< .001**
Avg. PA	**45.38 (15.32)**	**49.92 (14.77)**	**40.94 (14.65)**	**3.04**	**.003**
Avg. MDIS	**2.62 (.85)**	**2.36 (.80)**	**2.87 (.83)**	**3.11**	**.002**
Avg. Willpower	**3.52 (1.08)**	**3.76 (1.10)**	**3.29 (1.02)**	**2.17**	**.03**
Avg. Cause	2.52 (.96)	2.42 (1.02)	2.61 (.91)	1.00	.32
Avg. Judgment	2.70 (.98)	2.64 (.97)	2.77 (1.00)	.64	.53
Avg. Complexity	2.20 (.78)	2.15 (.71)	2.24 (.85)	.60	.55
Avg. Expression	2.32 (.86)	2.14 (.74)	2.49 (.95)	2.02	.05
Avg. Preference	3.16 (1.10)	3.36 (1.09)	2.97 (1.07)	1.79	.08
Avg. Control Behavior	2.89 (1.00)	2.71 (1.02)	3.07 (.94)	1.80	.08
Avg. Malleability	2.86 (.98)	2.80 (1.02)	2.91 (.94)	.54	.59
Avg. Uniqueness	**2.72 (.99)**	**2.48 (1.00)**	**2.96 (.92)**	**2.52**	**.01**
Avg. Longevity	**2.72 (1.03)**	**2.36 (.96)**	**3.07 (.98)**	**3.65**	**< .001**

Note. PAI-BOR = Personality Assessment Inventory-Borderline Features Scale; RR = response rate; NA = negative affect; PA = positive affect; MDIS = momentary distress intolerance. Bolded rows are statistically significant at $p < .05$.

Group Comparisons on Aggregated Data

Individual differences (i.e., PAI-BOR) and aggregated data across the week of EMA are reported in Table 2 both overall and by BPD group. The BPD features group reported higher homebase distress compared to the non-BPD group, although with no reported differences in homebase happiness. On the aggregated momentary variables, the BPD features group had higher negative affect, lower positive affect, higher momentary distress intolerance, and lower momentary willpower compared to the non-BPD group. The only differences between the two groups on aggregated momentary emotion beliefs was on uniqueness and longevity, where the borderline group reported greater beliefs that their emotions are unique and stronger beliefs that emotions last forever compared to the non-BPD group.

Stability and Fluctuation in Beliefs

Similarities and differences between baseline-assessed beliefs and aggregated state beliefs are presented in Table 3. All of the baseline beliefs were significantly and positively associated with the aggregated momentary belief assessing the same construct. Some of the baseline beliefs (beliefs about judgment, expression, preference of logic, beliefs that emotions control behavior, and beliefs about emotion longevity) were not significantly different from the aggregated momentary beliefs. However, people tended to report greater beliefs that emotions are not malleable during momentary reports when compared to baseline, yet lower beliefs that emotions are unique and lower beliefs that emotions should be "simple" (i.e., not complex) during momentary reports than when compared to baseline.

Analysis of the correlations (both between- and within-subject), ICCs, and MSSDs suggests that the beliefs have significant *between*-person variability (see Tables 4 and 5). The correlations (see Table 4) are considerably stronger between-person compared to within-person correlations, although it is also worth noting that most of the correlations are low to moderate, with all below .60 (and most below .40) except for the .81 between-person correlation between malleability and control behavior beliefs.

TABLE 3. Descriptive Information on Baseline and Momentary Beliefs

Belief	Baseline M (SD)	Avg. Momentary M (SD)	r	t test	p
Cause	2.28 (1.00)	2.52 (.96)	.37	**2.14**	**.04**
Judgment	2.84 (1.14)	2.70 (.98)	.68	1.69	.09
Complexity	2.44 (.98)	2.20 (.78)	.43	**2.47**	**.02**
Expression	2.37 (1.08)	2.32 (.86)	.71	.75	.46
Preference	3.28 (1.37)	3.16 (1.10)	.66	1.19	.25
Control Behavior	2.72 (1.29)	2.89 (1.00)	.50	1.44	.14
Malleability	2.39 (.99)	2.86 (.98)	41	**4.16**	**< .001**
Uniqueness	3.14 (1.19)	2.72 (.99)	.66	**4.62**	**< .001**
Longevity	2.71 (1.24)	2.72 (1.03)	.56	.15	.88

Note. Bolded rows are statistically significant at $p < .05$.

TABLE 4. Within and Between Correlations for Momentary Beliefs

Belief	1.	2.	3.	4.	5.	6.	7.	8.	9.
1. Cause	—	.01	.08**	.07**	−.11**	.04*	.07**	.04*	.12**
2. Judgment	−.14	—	.12**	.20**	−.02	−.02	.04	.12**	.01
3. Complexity	.10	.20*	—	.19**	.01	−.02	.02	.08**	−.03
4. Expression	−.06	.31**	.36**	—	−.02	−.06*	.02	.17**	−.04
5. Preference	−.25*	.19	.25*	.43**	—	−.07**	−.15**	.03	−.09**
6. Control Behavior	.57**	−.08	.08	−.10	−.32**	—	.18**	−.02	.12**
7. Malleability	.56**	−.12	−.05	−.22**	−.37**	.81**	—	.01	.14**
8. Uniqueness	.31**	.03	.22*	.16	.02	.08	.00	—	.07**
9. Longevity	.48**	.05	.08	.03	−.22*	.56**	.41**	.15	—

Note. Between-person correlations below the diagonal, within-person correlations above the diagonal. *p < .05. **p < .01.

The ICCs (see Table 5) were all over .50, with most at or above .70, which suggests that the brunt of the variability in beliefs is between people, rather than within-person. However, there was some within-person instability evident in the ICCs and was corroborated by the MSSD scores. The MSSD scores here are relatively consistent with MSSD scores of affective variables reported in prior studies, in the .50 to 1.00 range (Miller et al., 2009). An MSSD of zero would convey no changes in successive belief ratings over time.

We also examined MSSD and ICCs scores for the non-BPD and BPD features groups (see Table 5). Only the ICC for Cause was clearly different between the non-BPD and BPD groups (i.e., with nonoverlapping confidence intervals), where the BPD group showed greater within-person variability indicated by *lower* ICC scores. Even so, in general the BPD group tended to have lower ICC scores, suggesting somewhat greater variability within-person, which was consistent with the MSSD results, which found that the BPD

TABLE 5. Variability of the Beliefs by Borderline Features Group

Belief	ICC Overall [Lower CI; Upper CI]	ICC Non-borderline Features Group	ICC Borderline Features Group	MSSD Overall	MSSD Non-borderline Features Group M (SD)	MSSD Borderline Features Group M (SD)	t test	p
Cause	.71 [.65, .77]	.81 [.75, .87]	.61 [.52, .71]	.58 (.77)	**.39 (.41)**	**.70 (.82)**	2.39	.02
Judgment	.70 [.65, .77]	.75 [.67, .82]	.67 [.59, .76]	.62 (.90)	**.38 (.58)**	**.83 (1.08)**	2.54	.01
Complexity	.59 [.52, .66]	.55 [.45, .66]	.63 [.54, .73]	.65 (1.09)	.58 (1.22)	.65 (.79)	.36	.72
Expression	.70 [.64, .76]	.67 [.59, .76]	.71 [.63, .79]	.48 (.68)	.36 (.61)	.57 (.73)	1.48	.14
Preference	.77 [.72, .82]	.81 [.75, .87]	.71 [.62, .79]	.64 (1.03)	.45 (.78)	.76 (1.13)	1.55	.12
Control Behavior	.71 [.65, .77]	.73 [.65, .81]	.68 [.59, .77]	.67 (.83)	.59 (.85)	.74 (.81)	.87	.38
Malleability	.71 [.65, .77]	.77 [.70, .84]	.63 [.55, .74]	.69 (1.05)	**.43 (.50)**	**.94 (1.38)**	2.43	.02
Uniqueness	.68 [.62, .74]	.73 [.65, .81]	.59 [.50, .70]	.70 (.99)	**.43 (.59)**	**.89 (1.08)**	2.56	.01
Longevity	.74 [.69, .80]	.74 [.67, .82]	.69 [.61, .78]	1.02 (1.21)	.80 (1.09)	1.20 (1.30)	1.63	.11

Note. ICC = intraclass correlation coefficient; CI = confidence interval; MSSD = mean-squared successive difference.
Bolded rows are statistically significant at $p < .05$.

features group tended to exhibit more instability of beliefs (see Table 4). Specifically, the BPD features group had greater instability beliefs about emotion causes, judgment beliefs, malleability beliefs, and uniqueness beliefs compared to the non-BPD group.

Beliefs Predicted by Affect and Moderated by BPD Group

The role of negative and positive affect along with BPD group and interactions between BPD group and affect predicting momentary beliefs are presented in Table 6. In terms of BPD group main effects, these analyses had similar results to aggregated data at the person level (from Table 1); people in the BPD features group had stronger uniqueness beliefs and higher longevity beliefs compared to people in the non-BPD group but did not significantly differ on the other beliefs.

The majority of the beliefs (judgment, complexity, expression, preference, uniqueness, and longevity) were predicted by negative affect. For some of the beliefs, the influence of negative affect was helpful—people reported lower longevity beliefs and lower preferences for logic over emotion when feeling stronger negative emotion. However, the others showed greater increases in maladaptive beliefs alongside negative affect—beliefs that emotions are bad and destructive (judgment), beliefs that emotions should be simple (complexity), beliefs that emotions should be hidden from others (expression), beliefs that emotions cannot be changed (malleability), and beliefs that their emotions were different from others (uniqueness) were all stronger when negative affect was higher. In addition, negative affect interacted with BPD group to predict complexity, judgment, and uniqueness beliefs (see Figure 1). For the non-BPD group, negative affect predicted greater judgment ($B = .01$, $SE = .001$, $t = 8.12$, $p < .001$) and higher complexity (i.e., a stronger belief that emotions should not be complex; $B = .01$, $SE = .001$, $t = 5.16$, $p < .001$). Neither the relationship between negative affect and judgment ($B = .001$, $SE = .001$, $t = 1.42$, $p = .16$) nor that between negative affect and complexity ($B = .001$, $SE = .001$, $t = 1.31$, $p = .19$) was significant for the BPD features group. Finally, the relationship between negative affect and uniqueness beliefs was stronger for the non-BPD group ($B = .01$, $SE = .001$, $t = 6.89$, $p < .001$) than the BPD features group ($B = .001$, $SE = .001$, $t = 4.12$, $p < .19$).

In contrast, positive affect significantly predicted only malleability and uniqueness beliefs, whereby higher positive affect was associated with weaker beliefs that emotions cannot be changed (i.e., greater beliefs that emotions can be changed), but also stronger beliefs that their own emotions were different from others. However, BPD group interacted with positive affect to predict beliefs about cause and preference beliefs (see Figure 2). For the non-BPD group, greater positive affect was not associated with cause beliefs ($B = -.001$, $SE = .001$, $t = 1.34$, $p = .18$), whereas those in the BPD features group reported stronger beliefs that emotions come from out of nowhere in greater positive affect states ($B = .003$, $SE = .001$, $t = 3.17$, $p = .001$). In addition, for the BPD features group, greater positive affect was also associated with marginally weaker preferences for logic ($B = -.002$, $SE = .001$, $t = 1.82$, $p = .07$) and thus greater preferences for emotion, whereas for the non-BPD

TABLE 6. Negative Affect, Positive Affect, BPD Group, and Their Interactions Predicting Momentary Beliefs

Belief Outcome	Predictor	B (SE)	t	p
Cause	Negative Affect	.002 (.001)	1.72	.09
	Positive Affect	−.001 (.001)	−1.24	22
	BPD Group	.20 (.19)	1.02	.31
	NA × BPD	< .001	.42	.68
	PA × BPD	**−.002 (.001)**	**−3.05**	**.002**
Judgment	**Negative Affect**	**.01 (.001)**	**8.31**	**< .001**
	Positive Affect	< .001	.29	.77
	BPD Group	.12 (.20)	.58	.56
	NA × BPD	**.004 (.001)**	**5.11**	**< .001**
	PA × BPD	.001 (.001)	1.36	.17
Complexity	**Negative Affect**	**.007 (.001)**	**5.34**	**< .001**
	Positive Affect	< .001	.21	.83
	BPD Group	.09 (.16)	.60	.55
	NA × BPD	**.003 (.001)**	**3.14**	**.002**
	PA × BPD	.001 (.001)	1.09	.28
Expression	**Negative Affect**	**.009 (.001)**	**7.36**	**< .001**
	Positive Affect	**.002 (.001)**	**.01**	**.04**
	BPD Group	**.35 (.17)**	**2.03**	**.04**
	NA × BPD	−.002 (.001)	−1.25	.21
	PA × BPD	< .001	−.26	.80
Preference	**Negative Affect**	**−.004 (.001)**	**−.322**	**.001**
	Positive Affect	.002 (.001)	1.87	.06
	BPD Group	−.39 (.22)	−1.78	.08
	NA × BPD	−.001 (.002)	−1.19	.23
	PA × BPD	**.002 (.001)**	**2.34**	**.02**
Control Behavior	Negative Affect	.001 (.01)	1.02	.31
	Positive Affect	−.002 (.001)	1.98	.06
	BPD Group	.36 (.20)	1.79	.08
	NA × BPD	< .001	.04	.97
	PA × BPD	<.001	.60	.55
Malleability	Negative Affect	.002 (.001)	1.31	.20
	Positive Affect	**−.003 (.001)**	**−.2.57**	**.01**
	BPD Group	.10 (.20)	.53	.60
	NA × BPD	−.001 (.001)	−1.58	.11
	PA × BPD	< .001	.06	.95
Uniqueness	**Negative Affect**	**.01 (.001)**	**6.89**	**< .001**
	Positive Affect	**.002 (.001)**	**2.36**	**.02**
	BPD Group	**.49 (.19)**	**2.54**	**.01**
	NA × BPD	**−.001 (.001)**	**−2.02**	**.04**
	PA × BPD	<.001	−.63	.53
Longevity	**Negative Affect**	**−.006 (.001)**	**4.34**	**< .001**
	Positive Affect	−.002 (.001)	−1.80	.07
	BPD Group	**.70 (.20)**	**3.54**	**< .001**
	NA × BPD	< .001	−.30	.76
	PA × BPD	−.002 (.001)	−1.86	.06

Note. NA = negative affect; PA = positive affect; BPD = borderline features (1 = with borderline features; 0 = without). Bolded rows are statistically significant at $p < .05$.

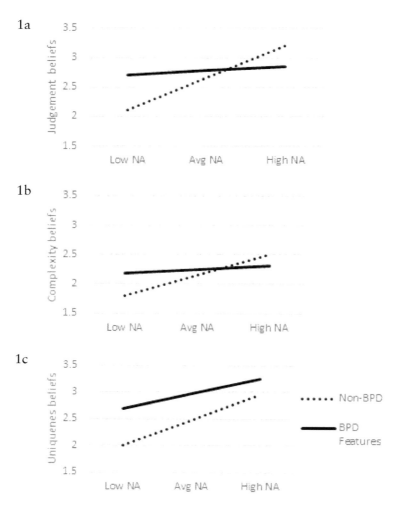

FIGURE 1. Interaction of negative affect and BPD group predicting Judgment, Complexity, and Uniqueness beliefs. 1a. Judgment Beliefs; 1b. Complexity Beliefs; 1c. Uniqueness Beliefs.

group greater positive affect was associated with greater preferences for logic ($B = .02$, $SE = .001$, $t = 2.06$, $p = .04$).

Beliefs about Emotion and Momentary Self-Efficacy

These models examined the role of beliefs in predicting momentary self-efficacy to tolerate distress (i.e., momentary distress intolerance) and to exert willpower. The results are presented in Table 7. Unsurprisingly, higher negative affect predicted both higher momentary distress intolerance and lower momentary willpower. When predicting momentary distress intolerance, there was

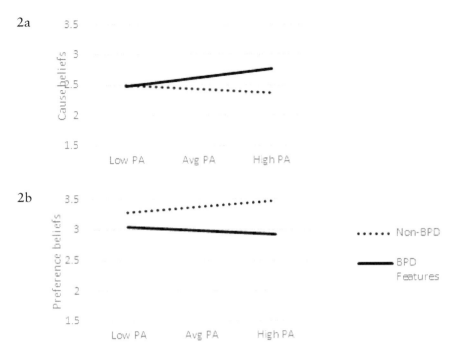

FIGURE 2. Interactions of positive affect and BPD group predicting Cause and Preference beliefs. 2a. Cause Beliefs; 2b. Preference Beliefs.

a main effect of complexity beliefs—stronger beliefs that emotions should be simple predicted greater momentary distress intolerance. In addition, there were several interactions between beliefs and BPD group for beliefs about judgment, preference, and behavioral control. In each of these, the relationship between the belief and momentary distress intolerance were significant only for people in the BPD features group (see Figure 3). Specifically, greater preferences for feeling over logic weres associated with greater distress intolerance for those with BPD features ($B = -.07$, $SE = .03$, $t = 2.34$, $p = .02$), but not for the non-BPD group ($B = .04$, $SE = .04$, $t = -1.07$, $p = .29$). Greater beliefs that emotions are bad and destructive (judgment beliefs; $B = .08$, $SE = .03$, $t = 3.24$, $p = .001$) and greater beliefs that emotions control behavior ($B = .11$, $SE = .03$, $t = 3.84$, $p < .001$) were associated with higher distress intolerance for those with BPD features, whereas neither judgment ($B = -.01$, $SE = .03$, $t = .38$, $p = .71$) nor behavior control beliefs ($B = .01$, $SE = .03$, $t = .43$, $p = .67$) were predictive of momentary distress intolerance for those in the non-BPD group.

For willpower, there were main effects of both uniqueness and complexity. The belief that one's own emotions are unique from other people's emotions predicted greater momentary willpower. Beliefs that emotions should be simple (i.e., not complex) predicted lower momentary willpower. This main effect was qualified by a significant interaction with BPD group, such that

TABLE 7. Emotion Beliefs and BPD Group and Their Interactions Predicting Momentary Distress Intolerance and Momentary Willpower, Controlling for Negative Affect

	Predictor	B (SE)	t	p
Momentary Distress Intolerance	**Negative Affect**	.03 (.01)	29.87	< .001
	BPD Group	.51 (.16)	3.10	.002
	Cause	.03 (.04)	.77	.44
	Judgment	−.01 (.04)	−.38	.71
	Complexity	.07 (.03)	2.25	.02
	Expression	.01 (.04)	.38	.71
	Preference	.06 (.04)	1.60	.11
	Behavior Control	.01 (.03)	.43	.67
	Malleability	.05 (.03)	1.45	.15
	Uniqueness	−.03 (.03)	−.84	.40
	Longevity	.05 (.03)	1.57	.12
	BPD × -Cause	−.10 (.04)	1.95	.05
	BPD × Judgment	.10 (.04)	2.24	.02
	BPD × Complexity	.02 (.04)	.60	.55
	BPD × Expression	−.02 (.05)	−.38	.70
	BPD × Preference	−.10 (.04)	−2.03	.04
	BPD × Behavior Control	.10 (.04)	2.41	.01
	BPD × Malleability	−.02 (.04)	−.41	.68
	BPD × Uniqueness	−.06 (.04)	−1.47	.14
	BPD × Longevity	.06 (.04)	1.30	.20
Willpower	**Negative Affect**	−.02 (.001)	−15.34	< .001
	BPD Group	−.47 (.21)	2.21	.03
	Cause	−.01 (.04)	−.29	.77
	Judgment	.01 (.04)	.34	.74
	Complexity	−.96 (.04)	−2.84	.004
	Expression	−.06 (.04)	−1.35	.17
	Preference	−.02 (.04)	−.51	.61
	Behavior Control	−.03 (.03)	−.51	.61
	Malleability	.02 (.04)	−.86	.39
	Uniqueness	.11 (.04)	2.90	.004
	Longevity	−.03 (.03)	−.77	.44
	BPD × Cause	.02 (.05)	.51	.61
	BPD × Judgment	−.08 (.05)	−1.65	.10
	BPD × Complexity	.14 (.05)	2.99	.003
	BPD × Expression	.04 (.05)	.82	.41
	BPD × Preference	.10 (.05)	2.04	.04
	BPD × Behavior Control	−.12 (.05)	−2.47	.01
	BPD × Malleability	−.05 (.05)	−1.16	.25
	BPD × Uniqueness	−.07 (.05)	−1.23	.22
	BPD × Longevity	−.07 (.05)	−1.48	.14

Note. BPD = borderline features (1 = with borderline features; 0 = without). Bolded rows are statistically significant at $p < .05$.

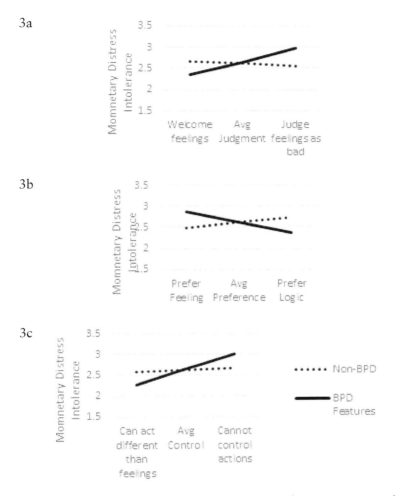

FIGURE 3. Interactions of beliefs and BPD group predicting momentary distress intolerance. 3a. Judgment Beliefs; 3b. Preference Beliefs; 3c. Control Behavior Beliefs.

the relationship between complexity beliefs and momentary willpower was driven by the non-BPD group (see Figure 4). For those without BPD symptoms, beliefs that emotions should be simple (i.e., not complex) predicted lower willpower ($B = -.10$, $SE = .03$, $t = 2.92$, $p = .003$), which was not evident for the BPD group ($B = .03$, $SE = .03$, $t = 1.08$, $p = .28$). There were also interactions between BPD group and both behavior control and preference. Specifically, greater beliefs that emotions control behavior predicted lower willpower for the BPD group ($B = -.14$, $SE = .03$, $t = 4.35$, $p < .001$) but not for the non-BPD group ($B = -.03$, $SE = .03$, $t = .85$, $p = .39$). Greater preferences for logic over feeling predicted greater willpower for the BPD group ($B = .08$, $SE = .03$, $t = 2.65$, $p = .008$) but not for the non-BPD group ($B = -.02$, $SE = .03$, $t = .51$, $p = .61$).

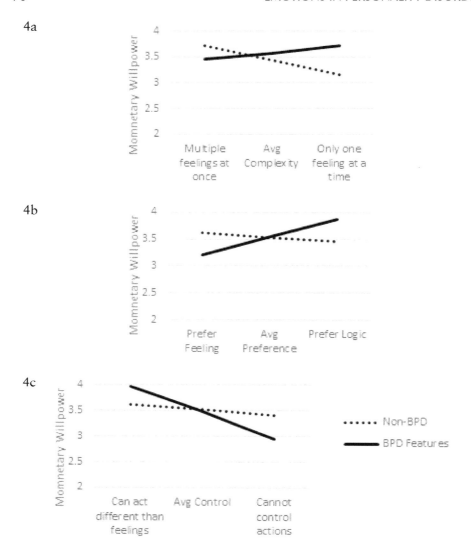

FIGURE 4. Interactions of beliefs and BPD group predicting momentary willpower. 4a. Complexity Beliefs; 4b. Preference Beliefs; 4c. Control Behavior Beliefs.

DISCUSSION

The goal of the current study was to determine *if* beliefs change across contexts (we thought they would) and to provide an initial examination of *for whom* beliefs change by explicitly comparing people with features of borderline personality to people without borderline features. We examined *in which emotional contexts* beliefs change by looking at positive and negative affect, and we examined the *implications* of emotion beliefs on momentary self-efficacy to tolerate distress and use willpower. Throughout, we also addressed the question of *which* beliefs change by looking at nine different beliefs about emotion measured multiple times per day over 1 week. Our overall conclusion is that yes, beliefs change, and in general more so for people with borderline features, but the relationships among beliefs, momentary emotion, and self-efficacy outcomes are complex and multifaceted.

Do Beliefs Change across Contexts?

Results from the current study support both stability *and* change. Evidence for stability comes from the relative consistency between the beliefs reported at the baseline lab session and the aggregated momentary beliefs (calculated over the entire week of EMA), paralleling recent work on personality traits which found that aggregated state personality data were fairly consistent with trait data (Rauthmann, Horstmann, & Sherman, 2019). Relatedly, we found fairly high intraclass correlations in the emotion beliefs, considerably higher than the typical EMA state data (often between .20 and .40; Bolger & Laurenceau, 2013). Most of our ICCs were around .70, suggesting that differences between people may be more prominent than differences within person over time in conceptualizing beliefs about emotion. These results support the construal of beliefs as primarily conveying schematic knowledge about the world (Burnette, O'Boyle, VanEpps, Pollack, & Finkel, 2013; Cervone, 2004; Leahy, 2002).

Beyond evidence of stability, there is also evidence for change. People reported greater beliefs that emotions "come from out of the blue," greater beliefs that emotions cannot be changed, *lower* beliefs that one's own emotions are different/unique from those of other people, and lower beliefs that emotions should be simple (i.e., experienced one-at-a-time) when assessed by moments compared to when they are assessed at a single time point at baseline. At the very least, these results suggest that a single belief assessment does not accurately capture the *level* of beliefs when aggregated over the moment. This in and of itself does not imply change, as it could reflect a reliability issue rather than a true index of instability. However, the rest of the results (i.e., ICCs, MSSDs) clearly suggest that beliefs *can* change over time. We thus turn our attention to the subsequent questions of *for whom* beliefs change, and in *which emotional contexts*.

For Whom Do Beliefs Change?

Although there are potentially many groups *for whom* beliefs about emotion may change over time, we chose to examine people with and without features of borderline personality disorder (BPD). It is worth noting that we are not trying to claim that BPD causes any of the effects reported here, because these are ultimately correlational data. Also, we recognize that people with BPD features tend to have comorbid symptoms of other mental health issues, particularly "distress" symptoms (e.g., worry, depression; Eaton et al., 2011), consistent with a hierarchical taxonomy of psychopathology (Kotov et al., 2017).

Our results confirm that people with BPD features report higher momentary negative affect and lower momentary positive affect, as well as higher reported difficulties with distress tolerance and lower momentary willpower compared to those without BPD features (Houben, Claes, Sleuwaegen, Berens, & Vansteelandt, 2018; Tomko et al., 2014). We also found that the BPD group reported that they walk around with higher levels of typical or "baseline" distress than the non-BPD group, consistent with the idea that people with BPD features have a more negative affective "homebase" (Ebner-Priemer et al., 2015).

Yet only significant differences on the beliefs themselves were on uniqueness and longevity—people with BPD features felt their emotions were more different from those of other people and more strongly endorsed the belief that emotions would last "forever." These endorsed beliefs are consistent with findings that people with BPD features experience emotions differently than others (Chu et al., 2016; Santangelo et al., 2014). The heightened longevity beliefs in particular are consistent with reports that people with BPD typically take longer to return to emotional baseline compared to healthy controls (Ebner-Priemer et al., 2015).

In terms of belief instability, our results confirm that those with BPD features had greater mean-squared successive difference (MSSD) scores (i.e., greater instability) on beliefs about identifying the cause of emotions, judgment beliefs (i.e., beliefs that emotions are bad and destructive), malleability beliefs, and uniqueness beliefs. The other belief MSSDs did not show statistically significant differences between the BPD features group and the non-BPD group. In sum, the results here are consistent with the notion that people with borderline features experience variability in self-focused thoughts over time (Kanske et al., 2016; Tolpin et al., 2004; Zeigler-Hill & Abraham, 2006).

Although we chose to focus on BPD features, we reiterate that BPD features are sometimes considered a proxy for general personality dysfunction (Hopwood, Good, & Morey, 2018), and that people with BPD diagnoses—as well as BPD features—also typically experience significant other psychopathology (e.g., depression, PTSD). For example, major depression has long been associated with shifts in cognition (Beck, Rush, Shaw, & Emery, 1979), and perhaps beliefs about emotion are influenced by depressive states. In this study, BPD features were used as a proxy for general dysfunctions in emotion dysregulation, emotional volatility, and interpersonal dysfunction, and any one of those component parts may be the central element to belief changeability, leaving the question of *for whom* beliefs change open for further scrutiny. Future work can continue to try to understand *for whom* beliefs change by examining different diagnostic groups or personality traits.

Which Beliefs Change with Emotion, and What Are The Implications?

To this point, we have mostly ignored the question about *which* beliefs change because we did not have any a priori predictions about specific beliefs. However, at this point it seems useful to examine the beliefs individually to understand which beliefs change in which types of emotional contexts.

Cause. Beliefs about the cause of emotions (i.e., "emotions come from out of the blue") was more unstable for people with BPD features, particularly in positive affect contexts. For people with BPD features, higher positive affect was associated with greater beliefs that emotions come from out of the blue. This is interesting because people with BPD diagnoses not only experience more negative affect (Ebner-Priemer et al., 2015) but also seem to interpret even ambiguous information with a negative lens (Baer et al., 2012). Perhaps those with BPD features find positive affect more confusing and less trustworthy.

Judgment. People reported stronger judgment beliefs (i.e., that negative emotions are "bad" and "destructive") along with higher reported negative affect, and the BPD features group showed greater variability in judgment beliefs compared to the non-BPD group. However, and somewhat surprisingly, the relationship between reported negative affect and judgment was higher for those without BPD features. Perhaps people with BPD features, who tend to experience greater "homebase" distress, find the experience of negative affect more familiar and are thus less likely to judge the experience of negative affect as worse while experiencing it.

We also found that people with BPD features experience more momentary distress intolerance alongside higher judgment beliefs, which was not evident for the non-BPD group. This finding suggests that in times where people with BPD features judge their emotions as "bad" that they are less able to tolerate their feelings. Importantly, this analysis controls for negative affect, suggesting that these shifts in momentary beliefs may be useful avenues of exploration in understanding how and when people with BPD features willingly encounter and "allow" their feelings (Linehan, 2015).

Complexity, Expression, and Preference. We address these three beliefs together because the preference for logic over emotion, the belief that emotions should be kept to the self (i.e., not expressed), and the belief that emotions should be simple (i.e., not complex or mixed) tend to be correlated (Veilleux, Chamberlain, et al., 2019), which we likewise found here at the between-subjects level. These three beliefs are about what people think emotion "should" be—a sense of "ideal" affect. These beliefs may be culturally loaded. Preference and expression beliefs are associated with gender; men tend to hold stronger preferences for logic and beliefs that suppressing the expression of emotion is valuable (Veilleux, Chamberlain, et al., 2019; Veilleux, Pollert, et al., 2019). We have not yet done any cross-cultural work on these beliefs, but it seems likely that these beliefs around "ideal" affect would be the beliefs to show the greatest cross-cultural variation. For example, people from other cultures with greater tolerance for contradiction (i.e., dialectical thinking; Spencer-Rodgers, Peng, & Wang, 2010) may hold lower beliefs that emotions "should" be simple.

In addition to the similarities in these three beliefs, there were also differences. Complexity beliefs were stronger alongside increased negative affect, particularly for the non-BPD group. Beliefs that emotions should not be expressed also increased alongside both negative and positive affect—this was essentially the only effect of expression beliefs in the entire study, which suggests that beliefs about expression may have more to do with how emotion is communicated rather than with how emotion is experienced (Kennedy-Moore & Watson, 2001). In contrast, preference beliefs *decreased* with higher negative affect and increased with positive affect for the non-BPD group, suggesting that the belief that logic is preferable may be reinforced during more positive affective states. Furthermore, when people in the BPD group experienced a shift toward preferring logic, they likewise reported greater willpower and lower distress intolerance. The tendency to feel more in control accompanying increased preferences for logic may reflect a shift toward "wise mind" (Linehan, 1993, 2015) and emphasizes the cognitive component to both distress intolerance and willpower; people are more self-efficacious when they feel more cognitively capable.

Behavior Control and Malleability. The belief that emotions cannot be changed and must run their course (called *malleability* here, recognizing that high scores reflect low malleability) and the belief that emotions control behavior are strongly correlated at the individual difference level (Veilleux et al., 2015). Yet these two beliefs show differences across the momentary outcomes, reflective of the fairly low correlations at the within-person level. Beliefs that emotions are not malleable demonstrated more variability over time for the BPD group and were weaker alongside increased positive affect; none of these effects were evident for the behavior control beliefs.

Uniqueness. The belief that one's own emotions are different from beliefs of others (e.g., "no one feels the way I do") is the only belief that clearly assesses one's *own* emotions; the other beliefs assess beliefs about emotions in general. Interestingly, uniqueness was the only belief to show increases alongside *both* positive and negative affect. When people feel more emotional, they tend to report that their emotions are more different from others, regardless of the valence of the emotion.

We also replicated prior work that stronger uniqueness beliefs tend to be associated with increased borderline symptoms (Veilleux, Chamberlain, et al., 2019), where those with BPD features reported stronger and more variable uniqueness beliefs. People with BPD often report significant emotion invalidation, being told that they are "too sensitive" or that their emotions are somehow inappropriate (Zielinski & Veilleux, 2018), which is likely associated with beliefs about emotions as unique. Uniqueness beliefs also likely shift based on relational contexts. If a person shares his or her emotion with someone else and receives validation or support (i.e., "I would feel the same way!"), a person's sense that his or her emotions are different from those of others is likely to decrease. Future work may want to look specifically at uniqueness beliefs in moments where others are present, and/or examine a person's perception of momentary emotion validation—these are likely important contexts for fluctuations in uniqueness beliefs.

Longevity. Beliefs that emotions last "forever" were clearly associated with BPD features, consistent with past work suggesting that longevity beliefs are one of the beliefs most linked to psychopathology (Veilleux, Chamberlain, et al., 2019; Veilleux, Pollert, et al., 2019). We also found that when negative affect was higher, people reported weaker beliefs that emotions would last "forever," perhaps because most people can likely recognize that a current emotion—even a strong one—is not likely to be permanent. Perhaps longevity beliefs drive fear of emotions more than the current emotion itself.

Beliefs Across Contexts. In sum, most of the beliefs assessed here do seem to shift based on emotional context. Some of the beliefs (malleability, cause) were more tied to positive affect, whereas others (judgment, longevity, behavior control) were more tied to negative affect, and others (uniqueness) were tied to both. Some of the beliefs moved alongside emotion more so for people with BPD features (cause), whereas other beliefs were predominant for those without BPD features (judgment, complexity, preference). Yet this does not answer the question of whether it *matters* if beliefs shift while people are experiencing stronger affective experiences. If someone's beliefs are rigid and never changing, particularly if those beliefs are skewed toward the maladaptive side, that is likely problematic. It is also likely problematic if someone's beliefs are so pliable that they shift rapidly in different situations; these individuals may not have a stable sense of themselves or the world. Both of these problems are consistent with identity issues often seen in personality pathology (Morey, 2017). Our hunch is that stable adaptive beliefs are likely the most psychologically healthy. If someone can experience a strong negative emotion and still believe that emotions are acceptable, that others can feel the same way, that emotions will last only a short while, and that it's beneficial to share emotions with others, the person's emotional life will likely be richer and more flexible, both of which are associated with greater emotional well-being (Aldao, Sheppes, & Gross, 2015; Quoidbach et al., 2014).

Role of Emotion Beliefs in Momentary Self-Efficacy

Beliefs about emotion also likely matter in terms of motivating self-direction. People with personality pathology (including BPD) tend to experience difficulties with setting and achieving goals, and they tend to conflate thought with action (Morey, 2017), which is consistent with the heightened impulsivity and difficulties with distress tolerance often found in people with BPD (Selby & Joiner, 2009; Tomko et al., 2014). In this study, when preference for emotion was stronger, when beliefs that negative emotions are "bad" were stronger, people with BPD features tended to experience greater perceptions that they couldn't handle their emotions (i.e., greater momentary distress intolerance). In addition, beliefs about behavior control such as believing it is difficult—if not impossible—to act opposite an emotion were associated with both higher momentary distress intolerance as well as lower momentary willpower. A shift in preference toward logic over emotion was associated with greater willpower and greater distress tolerance for people with BPD. These results suggests that for people with BPD features, beliefs about emotions may be associated with a susceptibility to dysfunctional self-beliefs, including the notion of the self as powerless and incapable (Baer et al., 2012), whereas the perception of the self as holding greater logical capacity, as evidenced by a shift in preference toward logic or "rational mind" (Linehan, 1993), seems to be associated increased self-efficacy capacity. Treatments for BPD often include teaching skills to help people tolerate intense emotional experiences without engaging in actions that will make the situation worse (Linehan, 2015). Engaging in these skills is likely more difficult when a person believes that emotions are "in control" of his or her actions; targeting these beliefs may be particularly important for helping people with BPD features to act effectively.

Beliefs about emotions influence momentary self-efficacy for people in general, not just those with BPD features. In this study, when people reported stronger uniqueness beliefs and stronger beliefs that emotions should be simple, they also reported greater capacities for exerting self-control, suggesting that feeling different from others may have unique motivational properties. Understanding the types of goal-directed behavior associated with these beliefs may be useful—exerting self-control to hold one's tongue in an argument serves a relational function, whereas exerting self-control to stay at work late to finish a project serves an achievement function.

Understanding the link between emotion beliefs and momentary self-efficacy is important because of the role self-efficacy serves in motivating behavior (Cervone, 2000). When people think they are *not* capable of doing a task, they will be less likely to try or more likely to give up if initial efforts are not successful. We note that in this study we did not assess actual engagement in willpower or behavioral efforts to tolerate emotions and thus we do not yet know about the repercussions of momentary self-efficacy. Future work could expand on this study to examine how perceptions of momentary self-efficacy to tolerate distress serve as an important link between beliefs about emotion and actual behavioral choices.

Limitations

As with any study, this study has limitations. First, our sample was only college students, and there is reason to believe that people who are older (who often differ in emotional goals compared to younger people; Carstensen et al., 1999) also tend to have different beliefs about emotion (Veilleux, Chamberlain, et al., 2019; Veilleux, Pollert, et al., 2019) and may likewise differ on emotion belief dynamics. Second, we recognize that we used a self-report assessment of BPD features rather than an actual diagnostic interview, and thus we are assessing "features" rather than "disorder," although prior work has validated the use of borderline screening measures in college students, including the measure we used for recruitment (Gardner & Qualter, 2009; Trull, 1995). Third, our use of an "extreme groups" sampling strategy (those above the recommended clinical cutoff of $T = 70$ and those with a T score of 50 or below) may inflate effect sizes compared to using the full dimensional score assessing borderline features (Fisher et al., 2020), and it also undermines current approaches like the Appendix Model of Personality Disorder (AMPD), which advocate for a dimensional approach to personality pathology (Widiger, 2011). Fourth, there are likely other beliefs about emotion we did not assess here (e.g., the belief that emotions are "contagious"; Savani, Kumar, Naidu, & Dweck, 2011). Fifth, the IBAE is still a fairly new measure of emotion beliefs and more work can be done on the IBAE to ensure that the anchors provided represent the opposite ends of each dimension, that they are clearly understood by participants, and that each dimension is unique.

Finally, and importantly, these are ultimately still correlational data. We found that beliefs about emotion were associated with emotion and momentary self-efficacy, but the data cannot show that emotions themselves cause changes in beliefs, or that changes in beliefs cause shifts in self-efficacy. This work thus paves the way for future experimental studies that can examine emotion beliefs as a function of induced emotion. In addition, manipulating people's beliefs about emotions and examining the role of beliefs in causing shifts in self-efficacy and subsequent behavior will also be important future steps. Self-efficacy is a strong predictor of behavior (Cervone, 2000), but it is important to understand if and how beliefs about emotion may *cause* behavioral choices (e.g., drinking to cope, emotional eating, engaging in interpersonal arguments) as well as the emotion regulation strategies that people choose to engage in. This is likely particularly salient for people with personality pathology. Alternatively, perhaps behavioral choices may serve as a substitute path for examining emotion beliefs; not everyone may have clear access to his or her beliefs. For example, if someone starts feeling an emotion and then makes active efforts to avoid or escape from that feeling, this would suggest that the person believes the emotion is "bad" or perhaps it will "last forever" if he or she does not try to escape. This person may self-report that he or she believes negative emotions are helpful and useful, but is that even possible if the person's behaviors suggest otherwise? These are questions ripe for future research.

CONCLUSION

Returning to our central opening point, the current study solidifies the notion that beliefs about emotions matter (Ford & Gross, 2018, 2019; Kneeland, Dovidio, et al., 2016) and extends that notion to confirm that beliefs matter for people with borderline features. This is the first study we are aware of to examine a fairly large set of beliefs about emotion dynamically using ecological momentary assessment. We conclude that although beliefs about emotion certainly vary at the individual difference level, beliefs also can change over time, and they can vary *with* both positive and negative affect. Understanding *for whom* beliefs change over time can help clinicians target beliefs as potential treatment goals and help foster a greater understanding of the differences in the dynamic relationships between cognition and affect that can occur across people. Finally, examining the *implications* of momentary shifts in emotion beliefs may help us understand the functions of emotion beliefs in prompting self-regulatory actions—whether helpful or otherwise—and continue to increase awareness of how momentary cognitions may dynamically shape our sense of self and the choices we make in our daily lives.

REFERENCES

Aldao, A., Sheppes, G., & Gross, J. J. (2015). Emotion regulation flexibility. *Cognitive Therapy and Research, 39,* 263–278. https://doi.org/10.1007/s10608-014-9662-4

Baer, R. A., Peters, J. R., Eisenlohr-Moul, T. A., Geiger, P. J., & Sauer, S. E. (2012). Emotion-related cognitive processes in borderline personality disorder: A review of the empirical literature. *Clinical Psychology Review, 32,* 359–369. https://doi.org/10.1016/j.cpr.2012.03.002

Bandura, A. (2001). Social cognitive theory: An agentic perspective. *Annual Review of Psychology, 52*(1), 1–26. https://doi.org/10.1146/annurev.psych.52.1.1

Beck, A. T., Rush, J. A., Shaw, B. F., & Emery, G. (1979). *Cognitive therapy of depression.* New York, NY: Guilford Press.

Bolger, N., & Laurenceau, J.-P. (2013). *Intensive longitudinal methods: An introduction to diary and experience sampling research.* New York, NY: Guilford Press.

Brantley, P. J., Waggoner, C. D., Jones, G. N., & Rappaport, N. B. (1987). A daily stress inventory: Development, reliability, and validity. *Journal of Behavioral Medicine, 10*(1), 61–74.

Burnette, J. L., O'Boyle, E. H., VanEpps, E. M., Pollack, J. M., & Finkel, E. J. (2013). Mind-sets matter: A meta-analytic review of implicit theories and self-regulation. *Psychological Bulletin, 139,* 655–701. https://doi.org/10.1037/a0029531

Carstensen, L. L., Isaacowitz, D. M., Charles, S. T., Prakash, R. S., De Leon, A. A., Patterson, B., ... Janssen, A. L. (1999). Taking time seriously. *American Psychologist, 54,* 165–181. https://doi.org/10.1037/0003-066X.54.3.165

Cervone, D. (2000). Thinking about self-efficacy. *Behavior Modification, 24*(1), 30–56. https://doi.org/10.1177/0145445500241002

Cervone, D. (2004). The architecture of personality. *Psychological Review, 111,* 183–204. https://doi.org/10.1037/0033-295X.111.1.183

Chu, C., Victor, S. E., & Klonsky, E. D. (2016). Characterizing positive and negative emotional experiences in young adults with borderline personality disorder symptoms. *Journal of Clinical Psychology, 72,* 956–965. https://doi.org/10.1002/jclp.22299

De Castella, K., Goldin, P., Jazaieri, H., Ziv, M., Dweck, C. S., & Gross, J. J. (2013). Beliefs about emotion: Links to emotion regulation, well-being, and psychological distress. *Basic and Applied Social Psychology, 35,* 497–505. https://doi.org/10.1080/01973533.2013.840632

De Castella, K., Platow, M. J., Tamir, M., & Gross, J. J. (2018). Beliefs about emotion: Implications for avoidance-based emotion regulation and psychological health. *Cognition and Emotion, 32,* 773–795. https://doi.org/10.1080/02699931.2017.1353485

Dixon-Gordon, K. L., Chapman, A. L., Lovasz, N., & Walters, K. (2011). Too upset to think: The interplay of borderline personality features, negative emotions, and social problem solving in the laboratory. *Personality Disorders: Theory, Research, and Treatment, 2,* 243–260. https://doi.org/10.1037/a0021799

Eaton, N. R., Krueger, R. F., Keyes, K. M., Skodol, A. E., Markon, K. E., Grant, B. F., & Hasin, D. S. (2011). Borderline personality disorder co-morbidity: Relationship to the internalizing-externalizing structure of common mental disorders. *Psychological Medicine, 41,* 1041–1050. https://doi.org/10.1017/S0033291710001662

Ebner-Priemer, U. W., Eid, M., Kleindienst, N., Stabenow, S., & Trull, T. J. (2009). Analytic strategies for understanding affective (in)stability and other dynamic processes in psychopathology. *Journal of Abnormal Psychology, 118,* 195–202. https://doi.org/10.1037/a0014868

Ebner-Priemer, U. W., Santangelo, P., Kleindienst, N., Tuerlinckx, F., Oravecz, Z., Verleysen, G., ... Kuppens, P. (2015). Unraveling affective dysregulation in borderline personality disorder: A theoretical model and empirical evidence. *Journal of Abnormal Psychology, 124*(1), 186–198. https://doi.org/10.1037/abn0000021

Edwards, E. R., & Wupperman, P. (2019). Research on emotional schemas: A review of findings and challenges. *Clinical Psychologist, 23,* 3–14. https://doi.org/10.1111/cp.12171

Fisher, J. E., Guha, A., Heller, W., & Miller, G. A. (2020). Extreme-groups designs in studies of dimensional phenomena: Advantages, caveats, and recommendations. *Journal of Abnormal Psychology, 129,* 14–20. https://doi.org/10.1037/abn0000480

Ford, B. Q., & Gross, J. J. (2018). Emotion regulation: Why beliefs matter. *Canadian Psychology, 59*(1), 1–14. https://doi.org/10.1037/cap0000142

Ford, B. Q., & Gross, J. J. (2019). Why beliefs about emotion matter: An emotion-regulation perspective. *Current Directions in Psychological Science, 28*(1), 74–81. https://doi.org/10.1177/0963721418806697

Gardner, K., & Qualter, P. (2009). Reliability and validity of three screening measures of borderline personality disorder in a nonclinical population. *Personality and Individual*

Differences, 46(5–6), 636–641. https://doi.org/10.1016/j.paid.2009.01.005

Goldschmidt, A. B., Engel, S. G., Wonderlich, S. A., Crosby, R. D., Peterson, C. B., Le Grange, D., . . . Mitchell, J. E. (2012). Momentary affect surrounding loss of control and overeating in obese adults with and without binge eating disorder. *Obesity, 20,* 1206–1211. https://doi.org/10.1038/oby.2011.286

Gutentag, T., Halperin, E., Porat, R., Bigman, Y. E., & Tamir, M. (2016). Successful emotion regulation requires both conviction and skill: Beliefs about the controllability of emotions, reappraisal, and regulation success. *Cognition and Emotion, 31*(6), 1–9. https://doi.org/10.1080/02699931.2016.1213704

Hopwood, C. J., Good, E. W., & Morey, L. C. (2018). Validity of the *DSM-5* Levels of Personality Functioning Scale–Self Report. *Journal of Personality Assessment, 100,* 650–659. https://doi.org/10.1080/00223891.2017.1420660

Houben, M., Claes, L., Sleuwaegen, E., Berens, A., & Vansteelandt, K. (2018). Emotional reactivity to appraisals in patients with a borderline personality disorder: A daily life study. *Borderline Personality Disorder and Emotion Dysregulation, 5*(1), 1–13. https://doi.org/10.1186/s40479-018-0095-7

Howell, R. T., Ksendzova, M., Nestingen, E., Yerahian, C., & Iyer, R. (2017). Your personality on a good day: How trait and state personality predict daily well-being. *Journal of Research in Personality, 69,* 250–263. https://doi.org/10.1016/j.jrp.2016.08.001

Kanske, P., Schulze, L., Dziobek, I., Scheibner, H., Roepke, S., & Singer, T. (2016). The wandering mind in borderline personality disorder: Instability in self- and other-related thoughts. *Psychiatry Research, 242,* 302–310. https://doi.org/10.1016/j.psychres.2016.05.060

Kennedy-Moore, E., & Watson, J. C. (2001). How and when does emotional expression help? *Review of General Psychology, 5,* 187–212. https://doi.org/10.1037//1089-2680.5.3.187

Kneeland, E. T., Dovidio, J. F., Joormann, J., & Clark, M. S. (2016). Emotion malleability beliefs, emotion regulation, and psychopathology: Integrating affective and clinical science. *Clinical Psychology Review, 45,* 81–88. https://doi.org/10.1016/j.cpr.2016.03.008

Kneeland, E. T., Nolen-Hoeksema, S., Dovidio, J. F., & Gruber, J. (2016). Beliefs about emotion's malleability influence state emotion regulation. *Motivation and Emotion, 40,* 740–749. https://doi.org/10.1007/s11031-016-9566-6

Kotov, R., Waszczuk, M. A., Krueger, R. F., Forbes, M. K., Watson, D., Clark, L. A., . . . Zimmerman, M. (2017). The Hierarchical Taxonomy of Psychopathology (HiTOP): A dimensional alternative to traditional nosologies. *Journal of Abnormal Psychology, 126,* 454–477. https://doi.org/10.1037/abn0000258

Kuppens, P., Oravecz, Z., & Tuerlinckx, F. (2010). Feelings change: Accounting for individual differences in the temporal dynamics of affect. *Journal of Personality and Social Psychology, 99,* 1042–1060. https://doi.org/10.1037/a0020962

Kuppens, P., & Verduyn, P. (2015). Looking at emotion regulation through the window of emotion dynamics. *Psychological Inquiry, 26,* 72–79. https://doi.org/10.1080/1047840X.2015.960505

Leahy, R. L. (2002). A model of emotional schemas. *Cognitive and Behavioral Practice, 9,* 177–190.

Leahy, R. L. (2015). *Emotional schema therapy.* New York, NY: Guilford Press.

Leahy, R. L. (2016). Emotional schema therapy: A meta-experiential model. *Australian Psychologist, 51*(2), 82–88. https://doi.org/10.1111/ap.12142

Leahy, R. L., Tirch, D. D., & Napolitano, L. A. (2011). *Emotion regulation in psychotherapy.* New York, NY: Guilford Press.

Linehan, M. M. (1993). *Cognitive behavioral therapy of borderline personality disorders.* New York, NY: Guilford Press.

Linehan, M. M. (2015). *DBT skills training manual* (2nd ed.). New York, NY: Guilford Press.

Manser, R., Cooper, M., & Trefusis, J. (2012). Beliefs about emotions as a metacognitive construct: Initial development of a self-report questionnaire measure and preliminary investigation in relation to emotion regulation. *Clinical Psychology and Psychotherapy, 19,* 235–246. https://doi.org/10.1002/cpp.745

Miller, D. J., Vachon, D. D., & Lynam, D. R. (2009). Neuroticism, negative affect, and negative affect instability: Establishing convergent and discriminant validity using ecological momentary assessment. *Personality and Individual Differences, 47,* 873–877. https://doi.org/10.1016/j.paid.2009.07.007

Morey, L. C. (1991). *Personality Assessment Inventory: Professional manual.* Odessa, FL: Psychological Assessment Resources.

Morey, L. C. (2017). Development and initial evaluation of a self-report scale development and initial evaluation of a self-report form of the *DSM-5* Level of Personality Functioning Scale. *Psychological Assessment, 29*(10), 1302–1308. https://doi.org/10.1037/pas0000450

Quoidbach, J., Gruber, J., Mikolajczak, M., Kogan, A., Kotsou, I., & Norton, M. I. (2014). Emodiversity and the emotional ecosystem. *Journal of Experimental Psychology: General, 143,* 2057–2066. https://doi.org/10.1037/a0038025

Rauthmann, J. F., Horstmann, K. T., & Sherman, R. A. (2019). Do self-reported traits and aggregated states capture the same thing? A nomological perspective on trait-state homomorphy. *Social Psychological and Personality Science, 10*, 596–611.

Santangelo, P., Bohus, M., & Ebner-Priemer, U. W. (2014). Ecological momentary assessment in borderline personality disorder: A review of recent findings and methodological challenges. *Journal of Personality Disorders, 28*, 555–576. https://doi.org/10.1521/pedi_2012_26_067

Savani, K., Kumar, S., Naidu, N. V. R., & Dweck, C. S. (2011). Beliefs about emotional residue: The idea that emotions leave a trace in the physical environment. *Journal of Personality and Social Psychology, 101*, 684–701. https://doi.org/10.1037/a0024102

Selby, E. A., & Joiner, T. E. (2009). Cascades of emotion: The emergence of borderline personality disorder from emotional and behavioral dysregulation. *Review of General Psychology, 13*, 219–229. https://doi.org/10.1037/a0015687

Shiffman, S., Gwaltney, C. J., Balabanis, M. H., Liu, K. S., Paty, J. A., Kassel, J. D., . . . Gnys, M. (2002). Immediate antecedents of cigarette smoking: An analysis from ecological momentary assessment. *Journal of Abnormal Psychology, 111*, 531–545. https://doi.org/10.1037//0021-843X.111.4.531

Shiffman, S., Stone, A. A., & Hufford, M. R. (2008). Ecological momentary assessment. *Annual Review of Clinical Psychology, 4*(1), 1–32. https://doi.org/10.1146/annurev.clinpsy.3.022806.091415

Spencer-Rodgers, J., Peng, K., & Wang, L. (2010). Dialecticism and the co-occurrence of positive and negative emotions across cultures. *Journal of Cross-Cultural Psychology, 41*(1), 109–115. https://doi.org/10.1177/0022022109349508

Spradlin, S. E. (2003). *Don't let emotions run your life: How dialectical behavior therapy can put you in control.* Oakland, CA: New Harbinger Publications.

Tamir, M., John, O. P., Srivastava, S., & Gross, J. J. (2007). Implicit theories of emotion: Affective and social outcomes across a major life transition. *Journal of Personality and Social Psychology, 92*, 731–744. https://doi.org/10.1037/0022-3514.92.4.731

Tolpin, L. H., Gunthert, K. C., Cohen, L. H., & O'Neill, S. C. (2004). Borderline personality features and instability of daily negative affect and self-esteem. *Journal of Personality, 72*, 111–137. https://doi.org/10.1111/j.0022-3506.2004.00258.x

Tomko, R. L., Solhan, M. B., Carpenter, R. W., Brown, W. C., Jahng, S., Wood, P. K., & Trull, T. J. (2014). Measuring impulsivity in daily life: The Momentary Impulsivity Scale. *Psychological Assessment, 26*, 339–349. https://doi.org/10.1037/a0035083

Trull, T. J. (1995). Borderline personality disorder features in nonclinical young adults: 1. Identification and validation. *Psychological Assessment, 7*, 33–41.

Trull, T. J., & Ebner-Priemer, U. (2013). Ambulatory assessment. *Annual Review of Clinical Psychology, 9*, 151–176. https://doi.org/10.1146/annurev-clinpsy-050212-185510

Trull, T. J., Useda, J. D., Conforti, K., & Doan, B.-T. (1997). Borderline personality disorder features in nonclinical young adults: 2. Two-year outcome. *Journal of Abnormal Psychology, 106*(2), 307–314. https://doi.org/10.1037//0021-843x.106.2.307

Veilleux, J. C., Chamberlain, K. D., Baker, D. E., & Warner, E. A. (2019, July 8). Disentangling beliefs about emotions from emotion schemas. *PsyArXiv.* https://doi.org/10.31234/osf.io/vxeck

Veilleux, J. C., Hill, M. A., Skinner, K. D., Pollert, G. A., Baker, D. E., & Spero, K. D. (2018). The dynamics of persisting through distress: Development of a momentary distress intolerance scale using ecological momentary assessment. *Psychological Assessment, 30*, 1468–1478. https://doi.org/10.1037/pas0000593

Veilleux, J. C., Pollert, G. A., Skinner, K. D., Chamberlain, K. D., Baker, D. E., & Hill, M. A. (2019, July 11). Individual beliefs about emotion and perceptions of belief stability are associated with emotion dysregulation, interpersonal emotional attributes and psychological flexibility. *PsyArXiv.* https://doi.org/10.31234/osf.io/kaubg

Veilleux, J. C., Salomaa, A., Shaver, J. A., Zielinski, M. J., & Pollert, G. A. (2015). Multidimensional assessment of beliefs about emotion: Development and validation of the Emotion and Regulation Beliefs Scale. *Assessment, 22*, 86–100. https://doi.org/10.1177/1073191114534883

Veilleux, J. C., Skinner, K. D., Baker, D. E., & Chamberlain, K. D. (2019). *The relationship between affect and momentary perceived willpower in daily life.* Unpublished manuscript.

Widiger, T. A. (2011). The DSM-5 dimensional model of personality disorder: Rationale and empirical support. *Journal of Personality Disorders, 25*, 222–234. https://doi.org/10.1521/pedi.2011.25.2.222

Wilson, R. E., Thompson, R. J., & Vazire, S. (2017). Are fluctuations in personality states more than fluctuations in affect? *Journal of Research in Personality, 69*, 110–123. https://doi.org/10.1016/j.jrp.2016.06.006

Yik, M., Russell, J. A., & Barrett, L. F. (1999). Structure of self-reported current affect:

Integration and beyond. *Journal of Personality and Social Psychology, 77*, 600–619.

Yoon, S., Dang, V., Mertz, J., & Rottenberg, J. (2018). Are attitudes towards emotions associated with depression? A conceptual and meta-analytic review. *Journal of Affective Disorders, 232*, 329–340. https://doi.org/10.1016/j.jad.2018.02.009

Zeigler-Hill, V., & Abraham, J. (2006). Borderline personality features: Instability of self-esteem and affect. *Journal of Social and Clinical Psychology, 25*, 668–687. https://doi.org/10.1521/jscp.2006.25.6.668

Zielinski, M. J., & Veilleux, J. C. (2018). The Perceived Invalidation of Emotion Scale (PIES): Development and psychometric properties of a novel measure of current emotion invalidation. *Psychological Assessment, 30*, 1454–1467. https://doi.org/10.1037/pas0000584

Emotional Dysregulation and Childhood Adversity in Borderline Personality Disorder

Emily R. Edwards, PhD, Nina L. J. Rose, MA,
Molly Gromatsky, PhD, Abigail Feinberg, BA, David Kimhy, PhD, John T. Doucette, PhD, Marianne Goodman, MD,
Margaret M. McClure, PhD, M. Mercedes Perez-Rodriguez, MD, PhD, Antonia S. New, MD, and Erin A. Hazlett, PhD

> Long-standing theories of borderline personality disorder (BPD) suggest that symptoms develop at least in part from childhood adversity. Emotion dysregulation may meaningfully mediate these effects. The current study examined three factors related to emotion dysregulation—alexithymia, affective lability, and impulsivity—as potential mediators of the relation between childhood adversity and BPD diagnosis in 101 individuals with BPD and 95 healthy controls. Path analysis compared three distinct models informed by the literature. Results supported a complex mediation model wherein (a) alexithymia partially mediated the relation of childhood adversity to affective lability and impulsivity; (b) affective lability mediated the relation of childhood adversity to BPD diagnosis; and (c) affective lability and impulsivity mediated the relation of alexithymia to BPD diagnosis. Findings suggest that affective lability and alexithymia are key to understanding the relationship between childhood adversity and BPD. Interventions specifically targeting affective lability, impulsivity, and alexithymia may be particularly useful for this population.
>
> *Keywords*: borderline personality disorder, abuse, alexithymia, impulsivity, affective lability

Borderline personality disorder (BPD) is a complex, often debilitating illness characterized by severe dysregulation in mood, behavior, cognition,

---

From Mental Health Research, Education, and Clinical Center (MIRECC VISN-2), James J. Peters VA Medical Center, Bronx, New York (E. R. E., N. L. J. R., M. Gromatsky, A. F., D. K., M. Goodman, E. A. H.); Department of Psychiatry, Icahn School of Medicine at Mount Sinai, New York, New York (N. L. J. R., A. F., D. K., M. Goodman, M. M. M., M. M. P.-R., A. S. N., E. A. H.); Department of Environmental Medicine and Public Health, Icahn School of Medicine at Mount Sinai (J. T. D.); and Department of Psychology, Fairfield University, Fairfield, Connecticut (M. M. M.).

This research was supported in part by the VA Advanced Psychology MIRECC Fellowship Program, the VISN-2 MIRECC, a VA Research Career Scientist Award to Dr. Hazlett (1 IK6 CX001738), and two VA Merit Awards to Dr. Hazlett (CX002093 and CX001451). The views expressed here are the authors' and do not necessarily represent the views of the Department of Veterans Affairs.

Address correspondence to Emily R. Edwards, James J. Peters VA Medical Center, 130 W. Kingsbridge Rd., Bronx, NY 10468. E-mail: emily.edwards@yale.edu

---

Originally published with the title "Alexithymia, Affective Lability, Impulsivity, and Childhood Adversity in Borderline Personality Disorder" in the *Journal of Personality Disorders*, Volume 35, Supplement A. ©2021 The Guilford Press.

and relationships (American Psychiatric Association, 2013). At least 75% of individuals with BPD attempt suicide, including approximately 10% who ultimately die by suicide (Black, Blum, Pfohl, & Hale, 2004). Enormous emotional distress and functional impairments associated with the disorder contribute to reduced productivity, severe impairments in social functioning, high utilization of mental health services, and disproportionate involvement with the criminal justice system (Comtois & Carmel, 2016; Conn et al., 2010; Gunderson et al., 2011; Samuels, 2011).

Reducing the burden of BPD on both society and the individual requires an accurate understanding of factors underlying BPD. Etiological theories suggest that borderline symptoms develop at least in part from experiences of childhood adversity (e.g., abuse, neglect, or disruptions in attachment, often occurring within the context of a relationship with a parent or caregiver). Linehan's biosocial theory, for example, proposes that borderline symptoms develop through a transaction between biological emotional vulnerabilities (i.e., high emotional sensitivity, high emotional reactivity, and slow return to emotional baseline) and an emotionally invalidating social environment (i.e., an environment that characterizes the person's internal experience as wrong, inappropriate, and/or unacceptable; Crowell, Beauchaine, & Linehan, 2009; Linehan, 1993). Similarly, the mentalization model of BPD suggests that early experiences of abuse and/or neglect by caregivers contribute to the development of maladaptive biological, behavioral, and emotional adaptations to avoid threat and abandonment (Fonagy & Luyten, 2009).[1]

Widespread empirical evidence has accumulated in support of these theories. A recent meta-analysis of nearly 100 studies suggests that individuals with BPD are 13.91 times more likely to report experiences of childhood adversity (e.g., abuse, neglect) than healthy controls and 3.15 times more likely to report such experiences than individuals with other psychiatric disorders (Porter et al., 2020). Similarly, higher severity of reported abuse is associated with greater severity of symptoms among individuals with BPD (Kaplan et al., 2016; Soloff, Lynch, & Kelly, 2002). Prospective analyses similarly suggest that experiences of child abuse and neglect increase the risk of subsequently developing borderline traits in adolescence and adulthood (Goodman & Yehuda, 2002; Johnson et al., 2001; Widom, Czaja, & Paris, 2009, but see Infurna et al., 2016). Despite this widespread evidence, however, comparatively little research has explored potential mediators to explain the relationship between trauma and BPD diagnosis.

Growing evidence suggests that emotion dysregulation may meaningfully mediate this relationship. Emotion dysregulation is a multifaceted construct, consisting of impairments in modulation, awareness, understanding, acceptance, and behavior subsequent to emotional arousal (Bridges, Denham, & Ganiban, 2004; Gratz & Roemer, 2004). It is commonly considered a core feature of BPD (Glenn & Klonsky, 2009; Linehan, 1993), and its development is closely associated with experiences of childhood adversity, particularly

---

1. Notably, although experiences of childhood adversity are commonly referenced in etiological theories of borderline personality development, research suggests that various factors contribute to such development. Genetic and biological effects, for example, play a key role in the development of various features associated with BPD (Amad, Ramoz, Thomas, Jardri, & Gorwood, 2014).

disrupted attachment (Calkins & Hill, 2007; Steele, Steele, & Croft, 2008). Recent research suggests that emotion dysregulation at least partially accounts for associations between childhood adversities and outcomes closely associated with BPD, including eating disorders, depression, and nonsuicidal self-injury (Burns, Fischer, Jackson, & Harding, 2012; Hopfinger, Berking, Bockting, & Ebert, 2016; Huh, Kim, Lee, & Chae, 2017; Jennissen, Holl, Mai, Wolff, & Barnow, 2016; Peh et al., 2017). Preliminary evidence from nonclinical samples (e.g., samples recruited from college or community settings rather than treatment settings) also suggests that emotion dysregulation may mediate associations between childhood adversity and borderline traits (Fossati et al., 2015; Kuo, Khoury, Meltcalfe, Fitzpatrick, & Goodwill, 2015). To date, however, these mediational relationships have not been investigated in samples diagnosed with BPD.

ALEXITHYMIA, AFFECTIVE LABILITY, AND IMPULSIVITY AS POTENTIAL MEDIATORS

Given the particularly salient role of emotion regulation within the relation between childhood adversity and psychopathology, it stands to reason that alexithymia, affective lability, and impulsivity—each of which conceptually overlaps with emotion regulation and is strongly associated with BPD—may similarly mediate the relation between childhood adversity and BPD. Alexithymia is a pervasive deficit in emotion processing and understanding characterized by difficulties in identifying and communicating emotional experiences and information (Bagby, Parker, & Taylor, 1994). Prior work, including work from our group, indicates that individuals with BPD have trouble accurately describing their emotional reactions and have more severe alexithymic trait severity compared with healthy controls (e.g., Hazlett et al., 2007; New et al., 2012). A more recent meta-analysis confirms a strong association between BPD and emotional awareness in studies comparing BPD with healthy controls (Derks, Westerhof, & Bohlmeijer, 2017). In addition, studies report associations between severity of alexithymia and BPD symptoms, including behavioral impulsivity, suicidality, and interpersonal dysfunction (Edwards & Wupperman, 2017; Kealy, Ogrodniczuk, Rice, & Oliffe, 2018; Spitzer, Siebel-Jurges, Barnow, Grabe, & Freyberger, 2005). Like BPD, disrupted child–caregiver relationships, interpersonal trauma, childhood adversity, and socialization experiences surrounding emotional expression, experience, and regulation are commonly theorized to contribute to alexithymic traits (Edwards, Micek, Mottarella, & Wupperman, 2017; Le, Berenbaum, & Raghavan, 2002; Thorberg, Young, Sullivan, & Lyvers, 2011). Some evidence also suggests that alexithymia is critical to the understanding of emotion dysregulation because it mediates the effects of trauma on other factors related to emotion dysregulation (e.g., distress intolerance; Fang & Chung, 2019; Gaher, Arens, & Shishido, 2015; Gaher, Hofman, Simons, & Hunsaker, 2013). Preliminary evidence suggests that this mediation effect may have especially notable implications for understanding borderline personality disorder. In a nonclinical sample of young adults, alexithymia, negative urgency, and distress tolerance mediated the association between trauma and borderline symptoms, with alexithymia mediating effects of trauma on negative urgency and distress tolerance (Gaher et al., 2013).

Individuals with BPD and/or significant emotion dysregulation also often experience their emotions as intense, unpredictable, and in need of avoidance (Holm & Severinsson, 2011; Kreisman & Straus, 2010; Linehan, 1993; Spodenkiewicz et al., 2013). Correspondingly, affective lability is common among persons with BPD (Reich, Zanarini, & Fitzmaurice, 2012; Silvers et al., 2016; Trull et al., 2008) and positively associated with BPD symptom severity (Links et al., 2007; Wedig et al., 2012). Like emotion dysregulation, childhood adversity likely contributes to the development of affective lability (Kim-Spoon, Cicchetti, & Rogosch, 2013; Shields & Cicchetti, 1998).

Lastly, individuals with BPD often display disrupted, impulsive cognitive and behavioral reactions, particularly in response to emotional experiences (American Psychiatric Association, 2013). Impulsivity is a core feature of BPD (Barker et al., 2015; Henry et al., 2001; Links, Heslegrave, & van Reekum, 1999) and manifests as poor self-control, nonplanning, behavioral reactivity, and/or inattention (Patton, Stanford, & Barratt, 1995). Like alexithymia and affective lability, impulsivity is closely associated with experiences of childhood adversity (Roy, 2005; Shin, Lee, Jeon, & Wills, 2015; Sujan, Humphreys, Ray, & Lee, 2014), although genetics also appears to be a strong contributor (Arce & Santisteban, 2006).

CURRENT RESEARCH

Previous research suggests that the relation between early interpersonal trauma and BPD may be at least partially explained by emotion dysregulation. However, reliance on nonclinical samples raises questions of clinical implications, and it remains unclear how alexithymia, affective lability, and impulsivity may also play a role in these mediational relationships. To address this gap in the literature, the current research examined alexithymia, affective lability, and impulsivity as potential mediators of the relation between childhood adversity and BPD diagnosis. Competing models, each informed by the literature, were compared using path analysis to best understand relations between these constructs. Consistent with previous research, we hypothesized:

1. Greater severities of alexithymia, affective lability, impulsivity, and childhood adversity would be associated with BPD diagnosis.
2. Alexithymia, affective lability, and impulsivity would each at least partially mediate relations between childhood adversity and BPD diagnosis.
3. Alexithymia would at least partially mediate effects of childhood adversity on affective lability and impulsivity.

METHOD

Participants

The sample included 196 individuals, including 101 with BPD and 95 healthy controls (HC) recruited as part of a larger program of research. Significant heterogeneity in age ($M = 35.19$, $SD = 11.28$, range = 18–65), race (45% White, 32% Black, 13% Asian, 6% Mixed Race), and years of education ($M = 14.93$, $SD = 2.76$, range = 3–24) were noted across the sample. Alexithymia data from a subset of these participants have been published elsewhere (e.g., New et al., 2012); nevertheless, the current study represents a novel analysis of such data by including different variables than those examined in previous work. See Table 1 for a summary of participant demographic information.

Participants were recruited through advertisements in local newspapers and Internet postings (e.g., Craigslist). To support recruitment of both individuals with BPD and HCs, multiple advertisements were used (e.g., advertisements noting difficulties with intense emotion targeted recruitment of individuals with BPD, whereas more generalized advertisements targeted HCs). Less than 10% of the individuals with BPD were recruited by referrals from the outpatient mental health clinics at Mount Sinai Hospital. All assessments were conducted at the Mood and Personality Research Program offices at Mount Sinai Hospital. All patients were free of any psychotropic medication for at least 2 weeks (6 weeks for fluoxetine) before the assessment, and most were never previously medicated. Exclusion criteria included history of schizophrenia or schizoaffective disorder, bipolar disorder type I, head trauma with loss of consciousness, neurological disease, organic mental syndrome, intellectual disability disorder, current substance use disorder (occurring within the past 3 months), or current major depressive episode (occurring within the past 3 months). Additional exclusion criteria for HC participants included personal history of any Axis I or personality disorder and first-degree family history of psychotic disorders.

MEASURES AND PROCEDURE

Diagnosis of Borderline Personality Disorder. All participants received a structured diagnostic interview administered by a clinical psychologist with expertise in evaluation of personality disorders using the Structured Clinical Interview for *DSM-IV* (SCID-IV; First, Spitzer, Gibbon, & Williams, 2002) and the Structured Interview for *DSM-IV* Personality (SIDP-IV; Pfohl, Blum, & Zimmerman, 1997). Our group has achieved an interrater reliability of $k = 0.80–0.81$ for the diagnosis of BPD (e.g., Goodman et al., 2014), as was true for the current sample.

Following the diagnostic interview, the participants completed the Childhood Trauma Questionnaire, the Toronto Alexithymia Scale-20, the Affective Lability Scale, and the Barratt Impulsiveness Scale as part of a larger study. Participants were provided monetary compensation for their time and travel. All procedures were approved by the Institutional Review Board at Icahn School of Medicine at Mount Sinai.

TABLE 1. Demographic and Clinical Measures

	Subjects With Borderline Personality Disorder (BPD) (n = 101)		Healthy Controls (n = 95)		
	M or n	SD or %	M or N	SD or %	Statistical Comparison
Age	34.35	11.31	34.25	11.32	$t(194) = .06, p = .95, d = 0.01$
Gender (female)	65	64.36%	55	57.89%	$\chi^2 (1) = 0.86, p = .35$
Race (minority)	54	53.47%	53	55.79%	$\chi^2 (1) = 0.11, p = .74$
Years of Education	14.13	2.68	15.83	2.58	$t(189) = -4.46, p < .01, d = 0.65$
CTQ	60.79	16.58	43.64	8.79	$t(194) = 8.97, p < .01, d = 1.29$
TAS-20	52.18	13.20	35.72	9.57	$t(194) = 9.94, p < .01, d = 1.43$
ALS	84.42	31.79	22.43	20.74	$t(183) = 15.53, p < .01, d = 2.31$
BIS	73.44	11.83	54.65	10.51	$t(194) = 11.73, p < .01, d = 1.68$

Note. CTQ = Childhood Trauma Questionnaire; TAS-20 = Toronto Alexithymia Scale-20; ALS = Affective Lability Scale; BIS = Barratt Impulsivity Scale.

Self-Report Measures. The Childhood Trauma Questionnaire-Short Form (CTQ-SF; Bernstein et al., 2003) was used to assess experiences of childhood adversity. The CTQ is a 28-item retrospective self-report assessment of physical abuse (e.g., "I was punished with a belt, a board, a cord, or some other hard object"), emotional abuse (e.g., "People in my family said hurtful or insulting things to me"), sexual abuse (e.g., "Someone tried to make me do sexual things or watch sexual things"), emotional neglect (e.g., "I felt loved"), and physical neglect (e.g., "I didn't have enough to eat") occurring during childhood. It has demonstrated strong test–retest reliability, internal consistency, convergent validity, and discriminant validity across samples (Bernstein et al., 1994; Scher, Stein, Asmundson, McCreary, & Forde, 2001). Internal reliability in the current sample was α = 0.87.

The Toronto Alexithymia Scale-20 (TAS-20; Bagby et al., 1994) was employed to assess alexithymia. Commonly considered the gold standard in alexithymia assessment (Kooiman, Spinhoven, & Trijsburg, 2002), this 20-item self-report questionnaire assesses the difficulties identifying feelings (e.g., "I am often confused about what emotion I am feeling"), difficulties describing feelings (e.g., "It is difficult for me to find the right words for my feelings"), and externally oriented thinking (e.g., "I prefer to analyze problems rather than just describe them") aspects of alexithymia. The TAS-20 has demonstrated strong concurrent and discriminant validity, test–retest reliability, and internal reliability across populations and contexts (Kooiman et al., 2002; Taylor, Bagby, & Parker, 2003). In the current sample, α = 0.89.

The Affective Lability Scale (ALS; Harvey, Greenberg, & Serper, 1989) was used to assess affective lability. The ALS is a 54-item self-report measure of rapidly shifting mood, focusing specifically on depression, elation, anxiety, and anger (e.g., "One minute I can be feeling OK and then I feel tense, jittery, and nervous"). It has demonstrated strong test–retest reliability, internal reliability, and construct validity in both clinical and nonclinical samples (Aas et al., 2015; Harvey et al., 1989). In the current sample, α = 0.98.

The Barratt Impulsiveness Scale (BIS-11; Patton et al., 1995) was used to examine impulsivity. This self-report questionnaire includes 30 items assessing attention, motor impulsiveness, self-control, cognitive complexity, perseverance, and cognitive instability (e.g., "I do things without thinking"). The BIS-11 is the most widely used self-report measure of impulsivity (Stanford et al., 2009). Across contexts and populations, it has demonstrated strong test–retest reliability, internal consistency, and convergent validity with other self-report measures (but not behavioral measures; Stanford et al., 2009). Internal reliability for the current sample was α = 0.91.

Statistical Analysis

Path analysis using the lavaan package for R (v 3.4.4; R Core Team, 2013) was then used to explore the potential mediating roles of alexithymia, affective lability, and impulsivity on the association between childhood adversity and BPD (to preserve statistical power, only scale total scores were used in analyses). Post hoc power analyses using G*Power (Faul, Erdfelder, Lang, & Buchner, 2007) suggested that the sample size provided adequate statistical power for regression analyses to detect medium-sized effects (1-β > 0.99, α = .05, effect size f^2 = 0.15). To best understand these potential relations, three models, each informed by the previous literature, were compared:

A. Consistent with correlational studies (e.g., Barker et al., 2015; Kaplan et al., 2016; New et al., 2012, Reich et al., 2012), Model A assessed childhood adversity, alexithymia, affective lability, and impulsivity independently predicting BPD with no mediating relationships.

B. Consistent with mediational analyses suggesting emotion dysregulation to mediate the relation of childhood adversity to psychopathology (e.g., Huh et al., 2017; Peh et al., 2017), Model B assessed alexithymia, affective lability, and impulsivity fully mediating the association between childhood adversity and BPD.

C. Consistent with research suggesting alexithymia to mediate the relation of childhood adversity to other factors associated with emotion dysregulation (e.g., Fang & Chung, 2018), Model C assessed affective lability and impulsivity fully mediating relations of childhood adversity on BPD, with alexithymia partially mediating relations of adversity to affective lability and impulsivity.

For each model, global and local fit statistics were analyzed to determine goodness of fit of the model to the data. Estimated indirect effects were also calculated to better understand potential mediating relationships. Lastly, chi-square difference tests were used to compare models and determine which model was a best fit to the data.

RESULTS

Consistent with common comorbidities of BPD, many participants with BPD also met criteria for a range of other psychiatric diagnoses. The most common comorbid diagnoses included intermittent explosive disorder ($n = 64$), major depressive disorder (past; most recent episode >3 months prior to study participation; $n = 39$), alcohol use disorder ($n = 37$), substance use disorder (past; no substance use diagnosis during the past 3 months; $n = 29$), and posttraumatic stress disorder ($n = 26$). Exploratory t tests and chi-square analyses suggested that participants with BPD and HCs were comparable in terms of age, gender, and race (all p values $\geq .35$). Participants with BPD had slightly less education than HCs, $t(189) = -4.46$, $p < .01$, $d = 0.65$. See Table 1 for a summary of these demographic comparisons. A multivariate ANOVA also suggested significant differences between participants with BPD versus HCs in study measures, Wilks's $\Lambda = 0.45$, $F(4, 180) = 66.08$, $p < .01$. Follow-up univariate analyses suggested that participants with BPD reported significantly more severe alexithymia, affective lability, impulsivity, and histories of early-life interpersonal trauma than HCs (all $ps < .01$, $ds = 1.29-2.31$; Table 1). Diagnostic tests suggested no notable violations of regression assumptions (i.e., linearity, normality of residuals, homoscedasticity, independence of residuals) and no significant instances of multicollinearity (all variance inflation factors (VIFs) < 2.75). Data missingness was minimal (1.15%); therefore, listwise deletion was used throughout analyses to account for missing data.

Path Analysis

Correlational analyses suggested strong associations between assessed aspects of emotion dysregulation (i.e., alexithymia, affective lability, and impulsivity; see Table 2). Path analysis using maximum likelihood estimation further explored these associations in accordance with the proposed models. Given group differences in education level, education level was included as a covariate in all analyses. Model A tested whether childhood adversity, alexithymia, affective lability, and impulsivity each independently predicted BPD diagnosis with no mediating relationships between variables. Consistent with hypotheses, global fit statistics suggested that this model was not a good fit to the data, $\chi^2(6, N = 196) = 367.45$, $p < .01$, CFI = 0.38, RMSEA = 0.55, 90% CI [0.51, 0.60], SRMR = 0.35. Local fit statistics similarly suggested that this model underestimated all associations between variables (correlation residuals = 0.09–0.69).

Model B tested a simple mediation model wherein alexithymia, affective lability, and impulsivity fully mediated the relation of childhood adversity to BPD diagnosis. Global fit statistics reflected only marginal improvement in comparison to Model A and suggested that Model B was also not a good fit to the data, $\chi^2(4, N = 196) = 203.32$, $p < .01$, CFI = 0.66, RMSEA = 0.50, 90% CI [0.45, 0.56], SRMR = 0.19. Local fit statistics suggested that Model B showed good fit with regard to childhood adversity (correlation residuals = 0.00–0.03), but underestimated associations between other variables (correlation residuals = 0.04–0.45). Estimated indirect effects suggested that both affective lability and impulsivity significantly mediated the relation of adversity to BPD diagnosis.

Lastly, Model C tested whether affective lability and impulsivity fully mediated the relation of childhood adversity to BPD diagnosis, with

TABLE 2. Correlation Statistics

	Childhood Adversity	Alexithymia	Affective Lability	Impulsivity
Childhood Adversity	—			
Alexithymia	.51 (< .01)	—		
Affective Lability	.58 (< .01)	.67 (< .01)	—	
Impulsivity	.44 (< .01)	.69 (< .01)	.74 (< .01)	—
n	196	196	185	196

alexithymia partially mediating the relations of adversity to affective lability and impulsivity. Global fit statistics reflected a notable improvement in model fit in comparison to Models A and B and suggested that Model C was a good fit to the data, $\chi^2(2, N = 196) = 2.51$, $p = .29$, CFI = 1.00, RMSEA = 0.04, 90% CI [0.00, 0.15], SRMR = 0.01. Local fit statistics also showed good fit at the local level (correlation residuals = 0.00–0.05). All paths were positive and statistically significant at $\alpha = .05$. The model accounted for 60% of the variance in BPD diagnosis, 53% in affective lability, 51% in impulsivity, and 25% in alexithymia. Estimated indirect effects suggested that alexithymia significantly mediated the relationship between childhood adversity and affective lability and between adversity and impulsivity; affective lability significantly mediated the relationship between adversity and BPD diagnosis and between alexithymia and BPD diagnosis; and impulsivity significantly mediated the relationship between alexithymia and BPD diagnosis. Impulsivity did not, however, significantly mediate the relationship between adversity and BPD diagnosis. See Figure 1 for a graphical representation of Model C and Table 3 for further information about model parameters and mediation analyses.

Model comparisons using chi-square difference tests suggested that Model C best fit the data of the current sample: comparing Model A to Model B, $\chi^2(2) = 164.13$, $p < .01$; comparing Model A to Model C, $\chi^2(4) = 364.94$, $p < .01$; comparing Model B to Model C, $\chi^2(2) = 200.81$, $p < .01$. See Table 3 for a summary of statistics for each model.

DISCUSSION

The main findings of this study are that (a) affective lability mediated the relation of childhood adversity to BPD diagnosis, and (b) alexithymia partially mediated the relation of childhood adversity to other aspects of emotion dysregulation. This is consistent with growing research suggesting that emotion dysregulation mediates the relation of childhood adversity to outcomes closely related to BPD and that alexithymia may play a notable role in these mediational relationships (e.g., Burns et al., 2012; Fossati et al., 2015; Gaher et al., 2013; Hopfinger et al., 2016; Huh et al., 2017; Jennissen et al., 2016; Kuo et al., 2015; Peh et al., 2017). Although childhood adversity is not the only factor contributing to the development of BPD (genetics also appears

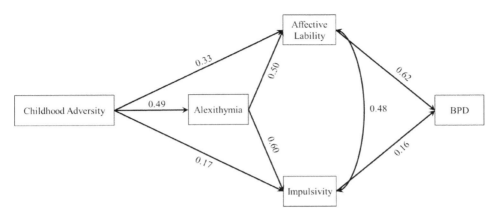

FIGURE 1. Model C. Due to the cross-sectional nature, results cannot be used to inform causal inference. Directionality of arrows in the figure is therefore purely theoretical and informed by previous research rather than by the current study design.

to play a key role; Amad et al., 2014), clarifying the nature of associations between childhood adversity and BPD could have direct implications for treatment. The current study is cross-sectional and therefore cannot inform causal models of this association; however, observed mediational relationships suggest that maintaining and/or developing healthy emotion regulation after childhood adversity may be key to minimizing the effects of adversity on the risk of developing BPD. Early interventions to develop and strengthen the emotion regulation of maltreated children may be helpful in this regard (e.g., Mazza, Dexter-Mazza, Miller, Rathus, & Murphy, 2016; Zenner, Herrnleben-Kurz, & Walach, 2014).

Results also suggest that affective lability may play a notable role in explaining these associations. Although all assessed factors (i.e., alexithymia, affective lability, and impulsivity) were significantly related to both a BPD diagnosis and severity of childhood adversity, affective lability showed notably stronger conditional associations with BPD and adversity in path analyses (see Table 3). By comparison, conditional effects of alexithymia and impulsivity were less pronounced. These findings suggest that affective lability may be more central to distinguishing individuals with BPD from healthy controls than disruptions in processing and/or responding to emotional experiences (i.e., alexithymia and impulsivity, respectively). This central function echoes characterizations of BPD as tending toward intense, labile emotional reactions (Holm & Severinsson, 2011; Kreisman & Straus, 2010; Linehan, 1993; Spodenkiewicz et al., 2013; Trull & Carpenter, 2014) and the emphasis of BPD-focused treatment programs on reducing emotional instability (e.g., Bateman & Fonagy, 2006; Linehan, 1993). Further research is needed to replicate and clarify this role of affective lability within the broader context of emotion dysregulation and BPD.

TABLE 3. Model Comparisons

	Model A (Independent Direct Effects)	Model B (Simple Mediation)	Model C (Complex Mediation)
Parameters			
CTQ → Diagnosis	$b = 0.10, p = .07$	—	—
TAS20 → Diagnosis	$b = 0.02, p = .67$	$b = 0.04, p = .47$	—
ALS → Diagnosis	$b = 0.64, p < .01$	$b = 0.64, p < .01$	$b = 0.62, p < .01$
BIS → Diagnosis	$b = 0.15, p < .01$	$b = 0.15, p < .01$	$b = 0.16, p = .02$
CTQ → TAS20	—	$b = 0.49, p < .01$	$b = 0.49, p < .01$
CTQ → ALS	—	$b = 0.58, p < .01$	$b = 0.33, p < .01$
CTQ → BIS	—	$b = 0.47, p < .01$	$b = 0.17, p < .01$
TAS20 → ALS	—	—	$b = 0.50, p < .01$
TAS20 → BIS	—	—	$b = 0.60, p < .01$
ALS → BIS	—	—	$b = 0.48, p < .01$
Variance Explained			
Diagnosis	$R^2 = 0.52, p < .01$	$R^2 = 0.56, p < .01$	$R^2 = 0.60, p < .01$
CTQ	$R^2 = 0.11, p < .01$	$R^2 = 0.11, p < .01$	$R^2 = 0.11, p < .01$
TAS20	$R^2 = 0.04, p < .01$	$R^2 = 0.25, p < .01$	$R^2 = 0.25, p < .01$
ALS	$R^2 = 0.15, p < .01$	$R^2 = 0.34, p < .01$	$R^2 = 0.53, p < .01$
BIS	$R^2 = 0.05, p < .01$	$R^2 = 0.24, p < .01$	$R^2 = 0.51, p < .01$
Mediation Effects			
TAS20 on CTQ → Diagnosis	—	$b = .02, p = .47$	—
ALS on CTQ → Diagnosis	—	$b = .37, p < .01$	$b = .20, p < .01$
BIS on CTQ → Diagnosis	—	$b = .07, p < .01$	$b = .03, p = .07$
TAS on CTQ → ALS	—	—	$b = .25, p < .01$
TAS on CTQ → BIS	—	—	$b = .29, p < .01$
ALS on TAS → Diagnosis	—	—	$b = .31, p < .01$
BIS on TAS → Diagnosis	—	—	$b = .09, p = .02$
Fit Statistics			
χ^2	$367.45, p < .01$	$203.32, p < .01$	$2.51, p = .29$
CFI	0.38	0.66	1.00
RMSEA	0.55	0.50	0.04
SRMR	0.35	0.19	0.01

Note. CTQ = Childhood Trauma Questionnaire; TAS20 = Toronto Alexithymia Scale-20; ALS = Affective Lability Scale; BIS = Barratt Impulsiveness Scale; CFI = comparative fit index; RMSEA = root-mean square error of approximation; SRMR = standardized root mean square residual.

The role of alexithymia in observed mediational relationships appears unique. Consistent with hypotheses and previous research (e.g., Fang & Chung, 2018; Gaher et al., 2013, 2015), alexithymia partially mediated the relation of childhood adversity to other factors related to emotion dysregulation. Fundamentally, alexithymia is an impairment in processing internal emotion cues (Lane, 2020). Because these cues provide necessary information to guide, control, and regulate behavior according to situational demands (Baumeister, Vohs, DeWall, & Zhang, 2007), restricted access to such information—as occurs in alexithymia—results in various forms of emotion dysregulation as observed in the current study. Findings suggest that histories of childhood adversity in BPD are associated with affective lability and impulsivity because of this restriction to emotional information. This may at least partially explain why treatments that increase attention to and processing of internal emotional cues (e.g., those based in mindfulness) are helpful for individuals with BPD. These mediation relationships are consistent with previous research, including models of subclinical borderline symptoms (e.g., Fang & Chung, 2018; Gaher et al., 2013, 2015). Such similarity in results across studies and populations suggests that the mediational role of alexithymia may extend across diagnoses and to both clinical and nonclinical populations. Findings are also consistent with evidence highlighting alexithymia as a necessary target in the treatment of trauma-related disorders and trauma-exposed persons (Berke et al., 2017; Hyer, Woods, & Boudewyns, 1991; O'Brien, Gaher, Pope, & Smiley, 2008; Zorzella, Muller, Cribbie, Bambrah, & Classen, 2020). Although treatment of alexithymia is often difficult for clinicians (O'Brien et al., 2008; Ogrodniczuk, Piper, & Joyce, 2011), recent findings suggest that psychoeducational and emotion-focused interventions may be effective in reducing alexithymic trait severity (Cameron, Ogrodniczuk, & Hadjipavlou, 2014; Edwards, Shivaji, & Wupperman, 2018; McMurran & Jinks, 2012). Given the role of alexithymia in mediating the relation of childhood adversity to other factors related to emotion dysregulation and, by extension, BPD, future research may examine the utility of alexithymia-focused interventions in the treatment and prevention of BPD.

Our results invite discussion about potential commonalities and differences between BPD and other types of psychopathology. For example, similar to persons with BPD, individuals with psychotic, depressive, eating, and trauma disorders display substantial degrees of alexithymia (Edwards, 2019; Kimhy et al., 2012; Kimhy et al., 2016; Li, Zhang, Guo, & Zhang, 2015; De Panfilis, Rabbaglio, Rossi, Zita, & Maggini, 2003) along with increased prevalence of childhood trauma and adversity (Brewin, Andrews, & Valentine, 2000; Hund & Espelage, 2006; Krabbendam, 2008; Mandelli, Petrelli, & Serretti, 2015; Morgan & Fisher, 2007; Thompson et al., 2009). Although preliminary, some evidence also suggests that alexithymia may play a similar mediating role for these disorders (Berenbaum, Valera, & Kerns, 2003; Güleç et al., 2013; Hund & Espelage, 2006; O'Brien et al., 2008). Future research should therefore investigate the extent to which results of the current study may also apply to other forms of psychopathology. It would be useful for future work to compare individuals with BPD to a clinical control group. Such comparisons could clarify the extent to which observed relationships are specific to BPD or reflective of broader patterns in psychopathology.

The current study has many strengths, most notably inclusion of a large sample of carefully diagnosed individuals with BPD. Nevertheless, results should be considered in light of a few methodological limitations. First, although the sample was prudently vetted to exclude potential confounding diagnoses, including active depression and a history of substance use, this vetting may also limit generalizability of findings to treatment settings. Typically, treatment-seeking individuals who meet criteria for BPD also meet criteria for at least three comorbid psychiatric conditions (Zimmerman & Mattia, 1999). Future research may therefore benefit from including a more diagnostically heterogeneous sample. Second, although etiological and developmental theories imply temporal order of effects, the current study used a cross-sectional design. Thus, findings cannot be used to imply or inform theories of temporal order or causal direction of observed effects. Relatedly, some evidence suggests that mediation analyses risk overestimating effects when using cross-sectional data (Maxwell & Cole, 2007). However, the present findings inform our understanding of the associations between childhood adversity, emotion regulation, and a BPD diagnosis. Longitudinal research is needed to investigate whether these models also reflect development of BPD in individuals over time. Third, strong reliance on use of self-report measures may have introduced issues of biased responding and/or method variance. Some research suggests that the limitations of self-report may be particularly salient for measures of trauma (Wilson & Keane, 2004) and alexithymia (Derks et al., 2017). Future research should therefore consider integrating laboratory, behavioral, and/or clinician-administered measures to provide a more complete perspective on mediating factors. Fourth, the study's sample size, while large for a clinical sample, limited statistical power to test more complex models, such as those controlling for potential confounds (e.g., comorbid conditions) or identifying latent variables that may be driving observed effects (e.g., different types of childhood trauma, subfactors of alexithymia, etc.). Future research may investigate these more complex models by employing larger samples. Lastly, the study focused on a narrow subset of constructs related to emotion dysregulation. It is likely that other factors, such as experiential avoidance, mindfulness, and use of specific regulation strategies, also play important roles in mediating the relation between trauma and BPD. Further research is needed to clarify these roles.

CONCLUSIONS

Theory and research have long suggested that experiences of childhood adversity are key to the development of BPD (e.g., Fonagy & Luyten, 2009; Linehan, 1993). However, only limited research has investigated potential mediating factors underlying the relation of childhood adversity to BPD. The current study replicates previous findings by offering further evidence to suggest a strong association between childhood adversity and BPD diagnosis. Extending previous findings, results also support a complex mediation model in which alexithymia, affective lability, and impulsivity mediate the association between childhood adversity and BPD, and alexithymia partially mediates the association of adversity to other aspects of emotion dysregulation.

REFERENCES

Aas, M., Pedersen, G., Henry, C., Bjella, T., Bellivier, F., Leboyer, M., . . . Etain, B. (2015). Psychometric properties of the Affective Lability Scale (54 and 18-Item Version) in patients with bipolar disorder, first-degree relatives, and healthy controls. *Journal of Affective Disorders, 172,* 375–380.

Amad, A., Ramoz, N., Thomas, P., Jardri, R., & Gorwood, P. (2014). Genetics of borderline personality disorder: Systematic review and proposal of an integrative model. *Neuroscience and Biobehavioral Reviews, 40,* 6–19.

American Psychiatric Association. (2013). *Diagnostic and statistical manual of mental disorders* (5th ed.). Arlington, VA: Author.

Arce, E., & Santisteban, C. (2006). Impulsivity: A review. *Psicothema, 18,* 213–220.

Bagby, R. M., Parker, J. D., & Taylor, G. J. (1994). The Twenty-Item Toronto Alexithymia Scale–I. Item selection and cross-validation of the factor structure. *Journal of Psychosomatic Research, 38,* 23–32.

Barker, V., Romaniuk, L., Cardinal, R. N., Pope, M., Nicol, K., & Hall, J. (2015). Impulsivity in borderline personality disorder. *Psychological Medicine, 45,* 1955–1964.

Bateman, A. W., & Fonagy, P. (2004). Mentalization-based treatment of BPD. *Journal of Personality Disorders, 18,* 36–51.

Baumeister, R. F., Vohs, K. D., DeWall, C. N., & Zhang, L. (2007). How emotion shapes behavior: Feedback, anticipation, and reflection, rather than direct causation. *Personality and Social Psychology Review, 11,* 167–203.

Berenbaum, H., Valera, E. M., & Kerns, J. G. (2003). Psychological trauma and schizotypal symptoms. *Schizophrenia Bulletin, 29,* 143–152.

Berke, D. S., Macdonald, A., Poole, G. M., Portnoy, G. A., McSheffrey, S., Creech, S. K., & Taft, C. T. (2017). Optimizing trauma-informed intervention for intimate partner violence in veterans: The role of alexithymia. *Behavior Research and Therapy, 97,* 222–229.

Bernstein, D. P., Stein, J. A., Newcomb, M. D., Walker, E., Pogge, D., Ahluvalia, T., . . . Zule, W. (2003). Development and validation of a brief screening version of the Childhood Trauma Questionnaire. *Child Abuse & Neglect, 27,* 169–190.

Black, D. W., Blum, N., Pfohl, B., & Hale, N. (2004). Suicidal behavior in borderline personality disorder: Prevalence, risk factors, prediction, and prevention. *Journal of Personality Disorders, 18,* 226–239.

Brewin, C. R., Andrews, B., & Valentine, J. D. (2000). Meta-analysis of risk factors for posttraumatic stress disorder in trauma-exposed adults. *Journal of Consulting and Clinical Psychology, 68,* 748–766.

Bridges, L. J., Denham, S. A., & Ganiban, J. M. (2004). Definitional issues in emotion regulation research. *Child Development, 75,* 340–345.

Burns, E. E., Fischer, S., Jackson, J. L., & Harding, H. G. (2012). Deficits in emotion regulation mediate the relationship between childhood abuse and later eating disorder symptoms. *Child Abuse and Neglect, 36,* 32–39.

Calkins, S. D., & Hill, A. (2007). Caregiver influences on emerging emotion regulation: Biological and environmental transactions in early development. In J. J. Gross (Ed.), *Handbook of emotion regulation* (pp. 229–248). New York, NY: Guilford Press.

Cameron, K., Ogrodniczuk, J., & Hadjipavlou, G. (2014). Changes in alexithymia following psychological intervention: A review. *Harvard Review of Psychiatry, 22,* 162–178.

Comtois, K. A., & Carmel, A. (2016). Borderline personality disorder and high utilization of inpatient psychiatric hospitalization: Concordance between research and clinical diagnosis. *Journal of Behavioral Health Services and Research, 43,* 272–280.

Conn, C., Warden, R., Stuewig, J., Kim, E. H., Harty, L., Hastings, M., & Tangney, J. P. (2010). Borderline personality disorder among jail inmates: How common and how distinct? *Corrections Compendium, 35*(4), 6–13.

Crowell, S. E., Beauchaine, T. P., & Linehan, M. M. (2009). A biosocial developmental model of borderline personality: Elaborating and extending Linehan's theory. *Psychological Bulletin, 135,* 495–510.

Derks, Y., Westerhof, G. J., & Bohlmeijer, E. T. (2017). A meta-analysis on the association between emotional awareness and borderline pathology. *Journal of Personality Disorders, 31,* 362–384.

De Panfilis, C., Rabbaglio, P., Rossi, C., Zita, G., & Maggini, C. (2003). Body image disturbance, parental bonding and alexithymia in patients with eating disorders. *Psychopathology, 36,* 239–246.

Edwards, E. (2019). Posttraumatic stress and alexithymia: A meta-analysis of presentation and severity. *Psychological Trauma: Theory, Research, Practice, and Policy.* Advance online publication. https://doi.org/10.1037/tra0000539

Edwards, E., Shivaji, S., & Wupperman, P. (2018). The Emotion Mapping Activity: Preliminary evaluation of a mindfulness-informed exercise to improve emotion labeling in alexithymic persons. *Scandinavian Journal of Psychology, 59,* 319–327.

Edwards, E. R., Micek, A., Mottarella, K., & Wupperman, P. (2017). Emotion ideology mediates effects of risk factors on alexithymia development. *Journal of Rational-Emotive and Cognitive-Behavior Therapy, 35,* 254–277.

Edwards, E. R., & Wupperman, P. (2017). Emotion regulation mediates effects of alexithymia and emotion differentiation on impulsive aggressive behavior. *Deviant Behavior, 38,* 1160–1171.

Fang, S., & Chung, M. C. (2019). The impact of past trauma on psychological distress among Chinese students: The roles of cognitive distortion and alexithymia. *Psychiatry Research, 271*, 136–143.

Faul, F., Erdfelder, E., Lang, A.-G., & Buchner, A. (2007). G*Power 3: A flexible statistical power analysis program for the social, behavioral, and biomedical sciences. *Behavior Research Methods, 39*, 175–191.

First, M. B., Spitzer, R. L., Gibbon, M. L., & Williams, J. B. W. (2002). *Structured Clinical Interview for DSM-IV-TR Axis I Disorders—Research version, non-patient edition.* New York, NY: Biometrics Research, New York State Psychiatric Institute.

Fonagy, P., & Luyten, P. (2009). A developmental, mentalization-based approach to the understanding and treatment of borderline personality disorder. *Developmental Psychopathology, 21*, 1355–1381.

Fossati, A., Gratz, K. L., Borroni, S., Maffei, C., Somma, A., & Carlotta, D. (2015). The relationship between childhood history of ADHD Symptoms and *DSM-IV* borderline personality disorder features among personality disordered outpatients: The moderating role of gender and the mediating roles of emotion dysregulation and impulsivity. *Comprehensive Psychiatry, 56*, 121–127.

Gaher, R. M., Arens, A. M., & Shishido, H. (2015). Alexithymia as a mediator between childhood maltreatment and impulsivity. *Stress Health, 31*, 274–280.

Gaher, R. M., Hofman, N. L., Simons, J. S., & Hunsaker, R. (2013). Emotion regulation deficits as mediators between trauma exposure and borderline symptoms. *Cognitive Therapy and Research, 37*, 466–475.

Glenn, C. R., & Klonsky, E. D. (2009). Emotion dysregulation as a core feature of borderline personality disorder. *Journal of Personality Disorders, 23*, 20–28.

Goodman, M., Carpenter, D., Tang, C. Y., Goldstein, K. E., Avedon, J., Fernandez, N., . . . Hazlett, E. A. (2014). Dialectical behavior therapy alters emotion regulation and amygdala activity in patients with borderline personality disorder. *Journal of Psychiatry Research, 57*, 108–116.

Goodman, M., & Yehuda, R. (2002). The relationship between psychological trauma and borderline personality disorder. *Psychiatric Annals, 32*, 337–345.

Gratz, K. L., & Roemer, L. (2004). Multidimensional assessment of emotion regulation and dysregulation: Development, factor structure, and initial validation of the Difficulties in Emotion Regulation Scale. *Journal of Psychopathology and Behavioral Assessment, 26*, 41–54.

Güleç, M. Y., Altintaş, M., İnanç, L., Bezgin, Ç. H., Koca, E. K., & Güleç, H. (2013). Effects of childhood trauma on somatization in major depressive disorder: The role of alexithymia. *Journal of Affective Disorders, 146*, 137–141.

Gunderson, J. G., Stout, R. L., McGlashan, T. H., Shea, M. T., Morey, L. C., Grilo, C. M., . . . Skodol, A. E. (2011). Ten-year course of borderline personality disorder: Psychopathology and function from the Collaborative Longitudinal Personality Disorders Study. *Archive of General Psychiatry, 68*, 827–837.

Harvey, P. D., Greenberg, B. R., & Serper, M. R. (1989). The Affective Lability Scales: Development, reliability, and validity. *Journal of Clinical Psychology, 45*, 786–793.

Hazlett, E. A., Speiser, L. J., Goodman, M., Roy, . . . M., Carrizal, M., Wynn, J. K., . . . New, A. S. (2007). Exaggerated affect-modulated startle during unpleasant stimuli in borderline personality disorder. *Biological Psychiatry, 62*, 250–255.

Henry, C., Mitropoulou, V., New, A. S., Koenigsberg, H. W., Silverman, J., & Siever, L. J. (2001). Affective instability and impulsivity in borderline personality and bipolar II disorders: Similarities and differences. *Journal of Psychiatry Research, 35*, 307–312.

Holm, A. L., & Severinsson, E. (2011). Struggling to recover by changing suicidal behaviour: Narratives from women with borderline personality disorder. *International Journal of Mental Health Nursing, 20*, 165–173.

Hopfinger, L., Berking, M., Bockting, C. L., & Ebert, D. D. (2016). Emotion regulation mediates the effect of childhood trauma on depression. *Journal of Affective Disorders, 198*, 189–197.

Huh, H. J., Kim, K. H., Lee, H. K., & Chae, J. H. (2017). The relationship between childhood trauma and the severity of adulthood depression and anxiety symptoms in a clinical sample: The mediating role of cognitive emotion regulation strategies. *Journal of Affective Disorders, 213*, 44–50.

Hund, A., & Espelage, D. (2006). Childhood emotional abuse and disordered eating among undergraduate females: Mediating influence of alexithymia and distress. *Child Abuse and Neglect, 30*, 393–407.

Hyer, L., Woods, M. G., & Boudewyns, P. A. (1991). PTSD and alexithymia—Importance of emotional clarification in treatment. *Psychotherapy (Chicago), 28*, 129–139.

Infurna, M. R., Brunner, R., Holz, B., Parzer, P., Giannone, F., Reichl, C., . . . Kaess, M. (2016). The specific role of childhood abuse, parental bonding, and family functioning in female adolescents with borderline personality disorder. *Journal of Personality Disorders, 30*, 177–192.

Jennissen, S., Holl, J., Mai, H., Wolff, S., & Barnow, S. (2016). Emotion dysregulation mediates the relationship between child maltreatment and psychopathology: A structural equation model. *Child Abuse and Neglect, 62*, 51–62.

Johnson, J. G., Cohen, P., Smailes, E. M., Skodol, A. E., Brown, J., & Oldham, J. M. (2001). Childhood verbal abuse and risk for personality disorders during adolescence and early adulthood. *Comprehensive Psychiatry, 42*, 16–23.

Kaplan, C., Tarlow, N., Stewart, J. G., Aguirre, B., Galen, G., & Auerbach, R. P. (2016). Borderline personality disorder in youth: The prospective impact of child abuse on non-suicidal self-injury and suicidality. *Comprehensive Psychiatry, 71*, 86–94.

Kealy, D., Ogrodniczuk, J. S., Rice, S. M., & Oliffe, J. L. (2018). Alexithymia, suicidal ideation and health-risk behaviours: A survey of Canadian men. *International Journal of Psychiatry in Clinical Practice, 22*, 77–79.

Kimhy, D., Gill, K. E., Brucato, G., Vakhrusheva, J., Arndt, L., Gross, J. J., & Girgis, R. R. (2016). The impact of emotion awareness and regulation on social functioning in individuals at clinical high risk for psychosis. *Psychological Medicine, 46*, 2907–2918.

Kimhy, D., Vakhrusheva, J., Jobson-Ahmed, L., Tarrier, N., Malaspina, D., & Gross, J. J. (2012). Emotion awareness and regulation in individuals with schizophrenia: Implications for social functioning. *Psychiatry Research, 200*(2-3), 193–201.

Kim-Spoon, J., Cicchetti, D., & Rogosch, F. A. (2013). A longitudinal study of emotion regulation, emotion lability-negativity, and internalizing symptomatology in maltreated and nonmaltreated children. *Child Development, 84*, 512–527.

Kooiman, C. G., Spinhoven, P., & Trijsburg, R. W. (2002). The assessment of alexithymia: A critical review of the literature and a psychometric study of the Toronto Alexithymia Scale-20. *Journal of Psychosomatic Research, 53*, 1083–1090.

Krabbendam, L. (2008) Childhood psychological trauma and psychosis. *Psychological Medicine, 38*, 1405–1408.

Kreisman, J. J., & Straus, H. (2010). *I hate you—Don't leave me: Understanding the borderline personality*. New York, NY: Penguin.

Kuo, J. R., Khoury, J. E., Metcalfe, R., Fitzpatrick, S., & Goodwill, A. (2015). An examination of the relationship between childhood emotional abuse and borderline personality disorder features: The role of difficulties with emotion regulation. *Child Abuse and Neglect, 39*, 147–155.

Lane, R. D. (2020). Alexithymia 3.0: Reimagining alexithymia from a medical perspective. *Biopsychosocial Medicine, 14*(21), 1–8.

Le, H. N., Berenbaum, H., & Raghavan, C. (2002). Culture and alexithymia: Mean levels, correlates, and the role of parental socialization of emotions. *Emotion, 2*, 341–360.

Li, S., Zhang, B., Guo, Y., & Zhang, J. (2015). The association between alexithymia as assessed by the 20-item Toronto Alexithymia Scale and depression: A meta-analysis. *Psychiatry Research, 227*, 1–9.

Linehan, M. M. (1993). *Cognitive behavioral treatment of borderline personality disorder*. New York, NY: Guilford Press.

Links, P. S., Eynan, R., Heisel, M. J., Barr, A., Korzekwa, M., McMain, S., & Ball, J. S. (2007). Affective instability and suicidal ideation and behavior in patients with borderline personality disorder. *Journal of Personality Disorders, 21*, 72–86.

Links, P. S., Heslegrave, R., & van Reekum, R. (1999). Impulsivity: Core aspect of borderline personality disorder. *Journal of Personality Disorders, 13*, 1–9.

Mandelli, L., Petrelli, C., & Serretti, A. (2015). The role of specific early trauma in adult depression: A meta-analysis of published literature: Childhood trauma and adult depression. *European Psychiatry, 30*, 665–680.

Maxwell, S. E., & Cole, D. A. (2007). Bias in cross-sectional analyses of longitudinal mediation. *Psychological Methods, 12*, 23–44.

Mazza, J. J., Dexter-Mazza, E. T., Miller, A. L., Rathus, J. H., & Murphy, H. E. (2016). *DBT skills in schools: Skills training for emotional problem solving for adolescents: DBT STEPS-A*. New York, NY: Guilford.

McMurran, M., & Jinks, M. (2012). Making your emotions work for you: A pilot brief intervention for alexithymia with personality-disordered offenders. *Personality and Mental Health, 6*, 45–49.

Morgan, C. & Fisher, H. (2007). Environment and schizophrenia: Environmental factors in schizophrenia: Childhood trauma—a critical review. *Schizophrenia Bulletin, 33*, 3–10.

New, A. S., Rot, M. A. H., Ripoll, L. H., Perez-Rodriguez, M. M., Lazarus, S., Zipursky, E., . . . Siever, L. J. (2012). Empathy and alexithymia in borderline personality disorder: Clinical and laboratory measures. *Journal of Personality Disorders, 26*, 660–675.

O'Brien, C., Gaher, R. M., Pope, C., & Smiley, P. (2008). Difficulty identifying feelings predicts the persistence of trauma symptoms in a sample of veterans who experienced military sexual trauma. *Journal of Nervous and Mental Disease, 196*, 252–255.

Ogrodniczuk, J. S., Piper, W. E., & Joyce, A. S. (2011). Effect of alexithymia on the process and outcome of psychotherapy: A programmatic review. *Psychiatry Research, 190*, 43–48.

Patton, J. H., Stanford, M. S., & Barratt, E. S. (1995). Factor structure of the Barratt Impulsiveness Scale. *Journal of Clinical Psychology, 51*, 768–774.

Peh, C. X., Shahwan, S., Fauziana, R., Mahesh, M. V., Sambasivam, R., Zhang, Y., . . . Subramaniam, M. (2017). Emotion dysregulation as a mechanism linking child maltreatment exposure and self-harm behaviors in adolescents. *Child Abuse and Neglect, 67*, 383–390.

Pfohl, B., Blum, N., & Zimmerman, M. (1997). *Structured Interview for DSM-IV Personality: SIDP-IV*. Washington, DC: American Psychiatric Publishing.

Porter, C., Palmier‐Claus, J., Branitsky, A., Mansell, W., Warwick, H., & Varese, F. (2020). Childhood adversity and borderline personality disorder: A meta‐analysis. *Acta Psychiatrica Scandinavica, 141*, 6–20.

R Core Team. (2013). R: A language and environment for statistical computing. R Foundation for Statistical Computing, Vienna, Austria. http://www.R-project.org/

Reich, D. B., Zanarini, M. C., & Fitzmaurice, G. (2012). Affective lability in bipolar disorder and borderline personality disorder. *Comprehensive Psychiatry, 53*, 230–237.

Roy, A. (2005). Childhood trauma and impulsivity: Possible relevance to suicidal behavior. *Archives of Suicide Research, 9*, 147–151.

Samuels, J. (2011). Personality disorders: Epidemiology and public health issues. *International Review of Psychiatry, 23*, 223–233.

Scher, C. D., Stein, M. B., Asmundson, G. J., McCreary, D. R., & Forde, D. R. (2001). The Childhood Trauma Questionnaire in a community sample: Psychometric properties and normative data. *Journal of Traumatic Stress, 14*, 843–857.

Shields, A., & Cicchetti, D. (1998). Reactive aggression among maltreated children: The contributions of attention and emotion dysregulation. *Journal of Clinical Child Psychology, 27*, 381–395.

Shin, S. H., Lee, S., Jeon, S. M., & Wills, T. A. (2015). Childhood emotional abuse, negative emotion-driven impulsivity, and alcohol use in young adulthood. *Child Abuse and Neglect, 50*, 94–103.

Silvers, J. A., Hubbard, A. D., Biggs, E., Shu, J., Fertuck, E., Chaudhury, S., . . . Stanley, B. (2016). Affective lability and difficulties with regulation are differentially associated with amygdala and prefrontal response in women with borderline personality disorder. *Psychiatry Research: Neuroimaging, 254*, 74–82.

Soloff, P. H., Lynch, K. G., & Kelly, T. M. (2002). Childhood abuse as a risk factor for suicidal behavior in borderline personality disorder. *Journal of Personality Disorders, 16*, 201–214.

Spitzer, C., Siebel-Jurges, U., Barnow, S., Grabe, H. J., & Freyberger, H. J. (2005). Alexithymia and interpersonal problems. *Psychotherapy and Psychosomatics, 74*, 240–246.

Spodenkiewicz, M., Speranza, M., Taieb, O., Pham-Scottez, A., Corcos, M., & Revah-Levy, A. (2013). Living from day to day: Qualitative study on borderline personality disorder in adolescence. *Journal of the Canadian Academy of Child and Adolescent Psychiatry, 22*, 282–289.

Stanford, M. S., Mathias, C. W., Dougherty, D. M., Lake, S. L., Anderson, N. E., & Patton, J. H. (2009). Fifty years of the Barratt Impulsiveness Scale: An update and review. *Personality and Individual Differences, 47*, 385–395.

Steele, H., Steele, M., & Croft, C. (2008). Early attachment predicts emotion recognition at 6 and 11 years old. *Attachment and Human Development, 10*, 379–393.

Sujan, A. C., Humphreys, K. L., Ray, L. A., & Lee, S. S. (2014). Differential association of child abuse with self-reported versus laboratory-based impulsivity and risk-taking in young adulthood. *Child Maltreatment, 19*(3–4), 145–155.

Taylor, G. J., Bagby, R. M., & Parker, J. D. (2003). The 20-Item Toronto Alexithymia Scale. IV. Reliability and factorial validity in different languages and cultures. *Journal of Psychosomatic Research, 55*, 277–283.

Thompson, J. L., Kelly, M., Kimhy, D., Harkavy-Friedman, J. M., Khan, S., Messinger, J. W., . . . Corcoran, C. (2009). Childhood trauma and prodromal symptoms among individuals at clinical high risk for psychosis. *Schizophrenia Research, 108*(1–3), 176–181.

Thorberg, F. A., Young, R. M., Sullivan, K. A., & Lyvers, M. (2011). Parental bonding and alexithymia: A meta-analysis. *European Psychiatry, 26*, 187–193.

Trull, T. J., & Carpenter, R. W. (2014). Components of emotion dysregulation in borderline personality. *Current Psychiatry Reports, 15*(1), 1–13.

Trull, T. J., Solhan, M. B., Tragesser, S. L., Jahng, S., Wood, P. K., Piasecki, T. M., & Watson, D. (2008). Affective instability: Measuring a core feature of borderline personality disorder with Ecological Momentary Assessment. *Journal of Abnormal Psychology, 117*, 647–661.

Wedig, M. M., Silverman, M. H., Frankenburg, F. R., Reich, D. B., Fitzmaurice, G., & Zanarini, M. C. (2012). Predictors of suicide attempts in patients with borderline personality disorder over 16 years of prospective follow-up. *Psychological Medicine, 42*, 2395–2404.

Widom, C. S., Czaja, S. J., & Paris, J. (2009). A prospective investigation of borderline personality disorder in abused and neglected children followed up into adulthood. *Journal of Personality Disorders, 23*, 433–446.

Wilson, J. P., & Keane, T. M. (Eds.). (2004). *Assessing psychological trauma and PTSD*. New York, NY: Guilford Press.

Zenner, C., Herrnleben-Kurz, S., & Walach, H. (2014). Mindfulness-based interventions in schools: A systematic review and meta-analysis. *Frontiers in Psychology, 5*, 603.

Zimmerman, M., & Mattia, J. I. (1999). Axis I diagnostic comorbidity and borderline personality disorder. *Comprehensive Psychiatry, 40*, 245–252.

Zorzella, K. P. M., Muller, R. T., Cribbie, R. A., Bambrah, V., & Classen, C. C. (2020). The role of alexithymia in trauma therapy outcomes: Examining improvements in PTSD, dissociation, and interpersonal problems. *Psychological Trauma, 12*, 20–28.

Shame in Borderline Personality Disorder: Meta-Analysis

Tzipi Buchman-Wildbaum, MA, Zsolt Unoka, MD, PhD,
Robert Dudas, MD, PhD, Gabriella Vizin, PhD,
Zsolt Demetrovics, PhD, and Mara J. Richman, PhD

> Shame has been found to be a core feature of borderline personality disorder (BPD). To date, there is no existing systematic review or meta-analysis examining shame in individuals with BPD as compared to healthy controls (HCs). A meta-analysis of 10 studies comparing reported shame in BPD patients to HCs was carried out. Demographic and clinical moderator variables were included to see if they have a relationship with the effect size. Results showed that those with BPD had more reported shame than healthy controls. In addition, in BPD patients and HCs, higher education level was related to lower reported shame. In HCs, it was found that those who were younger reported a higher level of shame. Finally, among BPD patients, there was a relationship between levels of reported shame and elevated PTSD symptomatology. These findings emphasize the clinical relevance of shame in individuals with BPD and the need to formulate psychotherapeutic strategies that target and decrease shame.
>
> *Keywords:* shame, borderline personality disorder, BPD, meta-analysis, review

Borderline personality disorder (BPD) is a debilitating mental disorder, known to carry serious consequences for the lives of those affected due to elevated levels of disease and death rates, especially from suicidality (Lieb, Zanarini, Schmahl, Linehan, & Bohus, 2004). Symptoms of BPD include nonsuicidal self-injury, suicidal ideations, increased occurrence of suicidal acts as compared to other disorders, impulsive behaviors, and an insecure sense of self. This pattern of instability is largely evident in social relations, in individuals' emotional state, and in the manner they perceive and evaluate themselves (American Psychiatric Association, 2013). Although shame is not a core criterion in the

---

From Doctoral School of Psychology, ELTE Eötvös Loránd University, Budapest, Hungary (T. B.-W.); Institute of Psychology, ELTE Eötvös Loránd University, Budapest, Hungary (T. B.-W., G. V., Z. D., M. J. R.); Department of Psychotherapy and Psychiatry, Semmelweis University, Budapest, Hungary (Z. U., M. J. R.); Department of Psychiatry, University of Cambridge, Cambridge, Older People's Mental Health Service, Cambridgeshire and Peterborough NHS Foundation Trust, Cambridge, and University of East Anglia, Norwich, UK (R. D.); Department of Clinical Psychology, Semmelweis University, Budapest, Hungary (G. V.); and Endeavor Psychology, Boston, Massachusetts (M. J. R.).

Address correspondence to Mara J. Richman, Endeavor Psychology, 10 Newbury St., Boston, MA 02116. E-mail: mjrichman7@gmail.com

---

Originally published in the *Journal of Personality Disorders*, Volume 35, Supplement A. ©2021 The Guilford Press.

diagnosis of BPD, accumulating evidence coming from both clinical practice (Lieb et al., 2004) and research (Brown, Comtois, & Linehan, 2002; Nathanson, 1994; Rüsch, Lieb, et al., 2007) has found that it is a core, dominant theme in those experiencing BPD symptoms.

Shame has been described as emotional difficulty as the result of a strict judgment of one's own personality as negative (e.g., having flaws or being damaged; Lewis, 1971; Tangney, Miller, Flicker, & Barlow, 1996). Shame is known to be an internal experience that occurs mainly when an individual perceives oneself as inferior. This devaluating perception often triggers efforts to minimize the risk of further harm, such as avoiding social situations and/or withdrawing while interacting with others (Gilbert, 1998). Although experienced internally, shame can be shown externally, such as through blushing, not engaging in conversation, and decreased eye contact, as well as in an immediate desire to move away from the situation producing shame (Gilbert, 1998; Tangney et al., 1996; Tracy & Matsumoto, 2008).

Current research has parsed shame into two types: (a) shame proneness, or the predisposition to feel shame in a diverse range of circumstances, and (b) state shame, or shame that is situation dependent and temporal (Rüsch, Lieb, et al., 2007). Considering this, studies have primarily utilized methods that distinguish between shame proneness and state shame, and between explicit and implicit shame (Rüsch, Lieb, et al., 2007; Unoka & Vizin, 2017). *Explicit shame* refers to shame that is conscious and evaluated by direct questioning, indicated by the individual in the form of self-report scales, whereas *implicit shame* refers to shameful responses that arise automatically, unconsciously, and are evaluated by indirect methods (Lewis, 1971; Ritter et al., 2014). Furthermore, certain studies have noted different types of shame, such as between characterological, behavioral, bodily shame and cognitive and existential shame (Scheel et al., 2014; Unoka & Vizin, 2017).

To date, shame has been identified by clinicians and researchers as one of the emotions most associated with persistent suicidal tendencies (i.e., self-harming acts, rage) and impulsive behaviors in people with BPD (Lester, 1997; Linehan, 1993a). Patients with BPD report significantly elevated levels of shame (e.g., proneness, state shame/explicit, and state shame/implicit among all different types of shame) relative to the general healthy population and as compared to other mental disorders (e.g., social phobia, major depression, narcissistic personality disorders, attention-deficit/hyperactivity disorder, and nonpersonality disorders; Ritter et al., 2014; Rüsch, Lieb, et al., 2007; Scheel et al., 2014; Unoka & Vizin, 2017). Moreover, shame in BPD has been found to have a negative association with a patient's self-esteem and quality of life, but a positive association with increased anger-hostility and unstable interpersonal relationships, a core symptom of those with BPD (Rüsch, Lieb, et al., 2007; Unoka & Vizin, 2017).

Although the clinical relevance of shame in BPD has been recognized by scientists and clinicians through research and practice, respectively, to date no quantitative review of the literature has been undertaken. Taking this into consideration, we present a meta-analysis of self-reported shame in those with BPD in order to elucidate its magnitude. Moderator variables such as age, gender, education, and other clinical variables were also assessed. In light of the literature, we hypothesized that BPD patients would report higher levels of shame than healthy controls (HCs) and that clinical and sociodemographic moderator variables would have an impact on reported shame in both BPD patients and HCs.

METHOD

Data Collection

Overall Literature Search. Our search was conducted using both PubMed and PsycINFO with the search terms "borderline personality disorder" OR "BPD" AND "Shame" AND "controls" OR "healthy controls." The search was limited to articles in English published between 1980 and March 2020 on human participants. In addition, we looked at the references from other articles and reviews on the same subject. The studies were discussed and reviewed by four of the authors (T.B.W, Zs.U., G.V., and M.J.R.) and had the following inclusion criteria: (a) used questionnaire or checklist measures of shame in those with BPD, (b) included a healthy comparison group, and (c) had statistical values that allowed the calculation of an effect size (Cohen's d). All potential shame questionnaires were considered because shame is many things and we looked at an aggregate variable.

The search initially generated 35 studies for potential inclusion in the study. Once we looked at these 35 studies, 10 articles were included (see Table 1). We excluded articles for the following reasons: (a) lack of control group ($n = 15$), (b) shame paradigm instead of a questionnaire ($n = 7$), and (c) lack of a BPD diagnosis but instead just BPD symptomatology ($n = 3$). We chose to do a meta-analysis with a control sample for a calculation of the Cohen's d, which we explain further in the Methods section.

Categorical Moderator Variables. We searched the articles for clinical moderator variables of comorbid mental health diagnoses (i.e., posttraumatic stress disorder [PTSD], major depressive disorder, anxiety disorder), drug use, medication use, and demographic variables of gender (i.e., percentage of sample that was male), education (i.e., mean years), mean age, and marital status. However, due to lack of inclusion of all these variables in all of the studies, we could include only gender, education, mean age, and comorbid PTSD as continuous moderator variables. When a significant effect for heterogeneity emerged, categorical moderator analysis of variables was performed. Mean age and gender (i.e., male sample percentage) were considered continuous moderator variables.

Data Analysis

Our meta-analysis was executed with Comprehensive Meta-Analysis, version 3.0 software (Borenstein, Hedges, Higgins, & Rothstein, 2005). Cohen's d values were calculated from the difference in scores between BPD patients and HCs on checklists and questionnaires of shame. The Cohen's d was analyzed

TABLE 1. Studies Used in the Meta-analysis

Study name	Shame scale(s)	Scale description
Bach, 2018	Young Schema Questionnaire 3-short form (YSQ-S3); defectiveness/shame	Measures shame as manifested by shameful beliefs about oneself
Dyer, 2015	Body Image Guilt and Shame Scale (BIGSS); shame	Measures shame related to body image
	Modification of the Survey of Body Areas (SBA); shame	Measures shame related to body areas
Gadassi, 2014	Experience Sampling Diary-mood assessment (response to social proximity) (from 0 to 4); shame	Measures shame in response to social proximity
Ritter et al., 2014	Experience of Shame Scale (ESS), German translation	Measures state shame
	Test of Self-Conscious Affect (TOSCA-3), German translation	Measures shame proneness based on individual's respond to different scenarios
Rüsch, Lieb, et al., 2007	Test of Self-Conscious Affect (TOSCA-3)-short version, German translation	Measures shame proneness based on individual's response to different scenarios
	Experience of Shame Scale (ESS), German translation	Measures state shame
Unoka & Vizin, 2017	Experience of Shame Scale (ESS)	Measures different manifestations of shame: character, behavioral, and bodily
Wiklander, 2012	Test of Self-Conscious Affect (TOSCA) first version; shame, Swedish translation	Measures shame proneness based on individual respond to different scenarios
Scheel et al., 2014	SHAME (a scale developed by the authors)	Measures different manifestations of shame: bodily, cognitive, and existential
Chan et al., 2005	Internalized Shame Scale (ISS)-total score	Measures trait shame
Mneimne, 2017	Experience Sampling Methodology–shame reports (from 1 to 6-extremely); average score for 14 days	Measures experience of shame in response to different interpersonal events

by using two means (BPD group and healthy comparison group) divided by standard deviations (SD). In accordance with Cohen (1988), the effect sizes were divided by level of magnitude of small ($d = 0.2$), medium ($d = 0.5$), or large ($d \geq 0.8$). The confidence intervals (CI) and z-transformations were done to see whether the Cohen's d values were statistically significant. In regard to homogeneity of the effect sizes across studies for shame, we used the Cochran Q-statistic (Hedges & Olkin, 1985). When we discovered heterogeneity with the Q-statistic, we used a random-effects model for a significant level of the mean effect sizes. To test publication bias, we used a funnel plot and the tests developed by Begg and Mazumdar (1994) and Egger, Smith, Schneider, and Minder (1997).

If there was heterogeneity, moderators were assessed with the Q-statistic. The demographic moderator variables (i.e., age, gender, education level, percent of sample with comorbid PTSD) were examined with meta-regression methods as continuous variables. Although our objective was to look at disparities between types of shame as well as the conclusions of different shame questionnaires, there was not enough data in the literature to provide calculation of the effects of such moderators.

RESULTS

Overall

Ten studies were included with 3,543 participants (HCs = 2,283, BPD = 1,260). Analysis of self-reported shame for the entire sample revealed a large effect size ($N = 3,543$, $d = 1.44$) with significant heterogeneity (Q_B [20] = 271.332, $p < .0001$). Considering that there was potential variability in the effect sizes within healthy and patient groups that were more than just a sampling error, moderator variable analyses were performed. The results are depicted in Figure 1.

Publication Bias

The funnel plot that was asymmetric and the Begg ($p = .0005$, 1-tailed) and Egger ($p = .0001$, 1-tailed) tests were significant, suggesting a possible "file drawer" problem. For the publication bias detection, fail-safe N calculation revealed that 4,970 "null" studies would need to be found and integrated in the meta-analysis to refute our findings. Therefore, the current findings represent the current literature of self-reported shame in individuals with BPD versus HCs.

Moderator Analyses

Demographic Variables. Moderator analysis by gender showed no significance in either the BPD sample ($Z = .28$, $p = .77$) or the HC group ($Z = .04$, $p = .96$). While the BPD group had no significance ($Z = .81$, $p = .41$), analysis showed

Shame in BPD

Study name	Effect Size within Study	Std diff in means	Standard error	Variance	Lower limit	Upper limit	Z-Value	p-Value
Boch 2018	A	2.006	0.173	0.030	1.667	2.344	11.626	0.000
Dyer 2015 a	A	1.855	0.332	0.110	1.205	2.506	5.591	0.000
Dyer 2015 a	B	1.850	0.332	0.110	1.200	2.500	5.579	0.000
Dyer 2015 b	A	2.229	0.365	0.133	1.514	2.944	6.108	0.000
Dyer 2015 b	B	2.007	0.352	0.124	1.318	2.696	5.709	0.000
Gadassi 2014	A	1.214	0.208	0.043	0.807	1.621	5.845	0.000
Ritter 2014	A	2.071	0.308	0.095	1.468	2.674	6.731	0.000
Ritter 2014	B	1.776	0.293	0.086	1.201	2.351	6.059	0.000
Rusch 2007	A	2.523	0.245	0.060	2.043	3.002	10.312	0.000
Rusch 2007	B	2.131	0.229	0.052	1.683	2.579	9.323	0.000
Unoka 2017	A	1.614	0.200	0.040	1.222	2.006	8.077	0.000
Unoka 2017	B	0.851	0.182	0.033	0.495	1.207	4.684	0.000
Unoka 2017	C	1.218	0.189	0.036	0.847	1.589	6.435	0.000
Wiklander 2012 a	A	1.104	0.133	0.018	0.843	1.365	8.291	0.000
Wiklander 2012 b	A	1.168	0.134	0.018	0.905	1.431	8.702	0.000
Scheel 2014	A	0.562	0.121	0.015	0.324	0.800	4.629	0.000
Scheel 2014	B	0.392	0.120	0.015	0.156	0.629	3.257	0.001
Scheel 2014	C	0.249	0.120	0.014	0.014	0.485	2.079	0.038
Scheel 2014	D	0.703	0.122	0.015	0.463	0.943	5.746	0.000
Chan 2005	A	2.534	0.293	0.086	1.959	3.108	8.642	0.000
Mneimne 2017	A	1.109	0.220	0.049	0.677	1.541	5.029	0.000
		1.444	0.150	0.022	1.151	1.738	9.646	0.000

FIGURE 1. Shame as depicted in a forest plot.
Effect sizes are depicted and subgroups within study are shown.

a significance for age in the HCs ($Z = -5.80$, $p = .0001$), showing that as age increased, self-reported shame decreased.

We found that as education level decreased, self-reported shame increased in both groups (BPD: $Z = -2.53$, $p = .01$; HC: $Z = -1.54$, $p = .02$). The mean education level was 13.5 years for patients with BPD and 15.6 for healthy controls.

Clinical Variables. Significance was found between comorbid PTSD and BPD ($Z = 2.48$, $p = .01$). As the percentage of those with comorbid PTSD in the sample increased, reported shame increased.

DISCUSSION

Our findings revealed a large overall effect size ($d = 1.44$) when looking at self-reported shame in those with BPD ased to healthy controls. Results revealed that individuals with BPD report considerably higher levels of shame levels than HCs. These findings are in accordance with the literature (Ritter et al., 2014; Rüsch, Lieb, et al., 2007; Scheel et al., 2014; Unoka & Vizin, 2017) and are the first to be validated in a meta-analysis.

The current study also found that several moderator variables influence shame in BPD, such as education and comorbid PTSD diagnosis. Age and gender, on the other hand, did not influence shame in BPD patients. These findings may stress the magnitude and understanding of shame as a widely experienced emotion not just parsed by gender. In the HC group too, gender was not found to influence shame, which is partially consistent with the literature, where some studies have reported gender differences (Ferguson & Crowley, 1997; Harvey, Gore, Frank, & Batres, 1997) and others have not (Harder, Cutler, & Rockart, 1992; Wright & O'Leary, 1989). As regards age in the HCs, we found that as age increased there was a significant impact on reported shame levels, which is in line with the human natural developmental pathway and with the maturity principle (Roberts, Wood, & Caspi, 2008). The maturity principle states that there is a positive development throughout life; that is, people are more likely to develop positive and socially contributing personal traits, such as pride, as a function of increasing age. On the contrary, maladaptive traits, such as shame, are expected to decline as individuals mature (Roberts et al., 2008). A study that tracked individuals' levels of shame over the life span provided further support for the maturity principle by finding decreasing shame levels with age (Orth, Robins, & Soto, 2010). Our results contribute to the developmental literature on BPD by showing that in the adult development of individuals with BPD, the "maturity principle" is not valid, at least in the area of shame (Cameron, Erisman, & Palm Reed, 2020; Roberts & Damian, 2019). On the other hand, in both groups, education was found to have a significant impact on shame. This contributes new insights to the existing body of literature because only a small number of studies have examined the relationship between shame and education. While one study (Hasson-Ohayon et al., 2012) that examined shame reported no association, another study (Vizin, Urbán, & Unoka, 2016) reported a positive relationship between education and shame in healthy and clinical samples. We hypothesize that the connection seen between education and higher levels of shame is due to one's social environment surrounding the individual while he or she is performing. This is in line with Stein and Kean (2000), who found that those who had social anxiety were more likely to have shame and therefore not be able to perform tasks in the education system (e.g., presentations, exams). Thus, we consider that the reason for shame is due to the social anxiety that could arise in those who have BPD symptoms in school. Further studies are needed to draw any conclusions about the association between shame and education; however, we would recommend looking at social anxiety disorder symptoms as a moderator variable or as a potential comorbidity.

Our findings supported our hypothesis that BPD patients are prone to report higher levels of shame than HCs. Researchers and clinicians have found that traumatic incidents, neglect, and distress experienced both in early years of life and as adults put individuals with BPD at risk of experiencing higher levels of shame and should all be regarded as important in the occurrence of shame in BPD (Linehan, 1993a). Furthermore, it is also evident that the severity of these occurrences, in particular the severity of both sexual and verbal (Vizin et al., 2016) abuse and of neglect, have a substantial role in the appearance of shame (Karan, Niesten, Frankenburg, Fitzmaurice, & Zanarini, 2014). Being sexually abused contains aspects of manipulation, which has a devastating influence on individuals, leading them to perceive themselves as weak, accompanied by feelings that produce pervasive shame (Karan et al., 2014). Being verbally abused is humiliating in itself and, if done by attachment figures, the shaming messages are internalized and the internalized other becomes shame producing (Unoka & Vizin, 2017). Being neglected emotionally may result in perceiving one's own desires and emotions as inappropriate in the eyes of others, which can also create feelings of shame (Karan et al., 2014). The association between trauma and shame was also supported by Chan, Hess, Whelton, and Yonge (2005), who found a significant positive relationship, not only among patients with a BPD diagnosis but also among those without BPD. Taking into account that sexual abuse of women with BPD is more prevalent than in the general population (about 62.4%; Zanarini et al., 2002) can be informative in understanding the high prevalence of shame in individuals with BPD.

The high prevalence of shame among BPD patients can also be explained by the etiology of BPD itself. While a range of theories supply different explanatory frameworks for the development of BPD, they all agree that shame proneness is an inherent component of the disorder. The biosocial model posits an interaction between individuals' elevated emotional susceptibility and the impact of being raised in a neglecting and invalidating environment, which is responsible for the appearance of BPD symptoms (Linehan, 1993a). The reason for this is that in a harsh environment, a child's negative emotions are criticized and perceived as a source of shame. An even more damaging process occurs when children begin to invalidate their own emotions, leading them to feel ashamed of their own emotional expressions. This has a long-lasting effect, resulting in high shame proneness in adult life (Linehan, 1993a).

Enduring feelings of shame can be the result of the mutual impact of traumatic incidents with neglect and judgmental interactions occurring in one's close environment early in life, and personal traits connected to danger-related bodily systems, which will all determine the magnitude of reaction to these negative incidents (Andrews, Qian, & Valentine, 2002; Mills, 2005). The impact of these incidents facilitates the creation of early maladaptive schemas (Young, Klosko, & Weishaar, 2003), which play a fundamental role in an individual's identity structure (Pinto-Gouveia & Matos, 2011; Tomkins, 1963; Young et al., 2003). Moreover, object relations theory (Kernberg, 1984) explains the centrality of shame proneness in the presentation of a BPD diagnosis with particularly negative and split self-representations of individuals with BPD, which are absent from any constructive or favorable self-representations. Supporting evidence come from studies comparing shame levels in different diagnoses; these studies report significantly higher levels of shame experienced by individuals diagnosed with BPD than individuals diagnosed with other affective disorders (Rüsch, Lieb, et al., 2007; Scheel et al., 2014). Shame levels in the face of negative affect have also been noted throughout the literature as significantly higher among the BPD group (Jacob et al., 2009). Moreover, in contrast to other negative emotions, the impact of shame specifically (when generated by the researchers) persists for a longer period of time among the BPD group than among the other diagnostic groups (Gratz, Rosenthal, Tull, Lejuez, & Gunderson, 2010). The perception that BPD by itself is characterized by amplified feelings of shame is reinforced and validated by the results of the current study comparing BPD patients to healthy controls.

The moderator analysis also provided essential insight into the current body of research regarding shame and BPD by targeting education as an important factor, because BPD patients with lower educational levels experienced significantly greater shame. This finding might contribute to the detection of patients who are specifically at risk and prone to more intense feelings of shame. Considering this, a more fitting psychotherapeutic intervention can be developed. Identification of patients who are prone to shame is important especially in the light of the findings. That is, higher shame levels were found among BPD patients who also suffer from PTSD. It has already been found that PTSD is associated with shame (Andrews, Brewin, Rose, & Kirk, 2000), and from Andrews et al.'s study, it seems that the comorbidity of BPD and PTSD is especially problematic.

The role of PTSD in the study results can be better understood through the role of shame in the etiology of PTSD. Shame is known to be a common reaction to trauma (Dahl, 1989) and a mediator between childhood abuse, trauma, and psychopathology later in life (Andrews, 1995, 1997). Shame is known to be a response related to defeat and submission, which is often involved in abuse and attack. More specifically, studies have found shame to be related to biological reactions (which were suggested to be rooted in the social humiliation involved in trauma) that can provoke fundamental biopsychosocial symptoms of PTSD (Tangney, Stuewig, & Mashek, 2007). Furthermore, the experience of shame is known to prevent integration of memory of the trauma into one's life story and identity and as a result impedes recovery (Feiring, Taska, & Lewis, 1996; Sippel & Marshall, 2011; Wilson, Drozdek, & Turkovic, 2006). The impact of shame is also known to be significant in chronic traumatic exposures (Herman, 1992). Moreover, there is substantial support for the association between higher shame and PTSD (Saraiya & Lopez-Castro, 2016). The study's result of the higher shame levels among BPD patients with comorbid PTSD further supports the notion regarding the association between shame and PTSD, especially because the study has been conducted among populations with a high prevalence of trauma. As such, it suggests an extra element of shame and suffering for BPD patients who also cope with PTSD. Thus, it also stresses the need for further research about shame among this group and its association and pathways to additional psychopathology. Nevertheless, the findings are meaningful on their own because they provide further support for the manifestation of PTSD in BPD and the key role of maladaptive emotions (Bolton, Mueser, & Rosenberg, 2006), especially because previous studies conducted among patients with BPD have not found such associations (Rüsch, Corrigan, et al., 2007).

Some studies report that BPD symptomatology decreases with age (Paris, Brown, & Nowlis, 1987; Stone, 2001), suggesting that some symptoms "burn out," that is, people learn how to live with them as they mature (Stevenson, Meares, & Comerford, 2003). In light of these studies, it is interesting to find that shame in our sample did not decrease. This finding might provide further support for studies that would examine individuals who experience a significant improvement in BPD symptoms, which represent a more acute manifestation of the disorder such as impulsivity, while temperamental symptoms such as anger have been found to be more persistent and long lasting (Zanarini et al., 2007). Considering the negative impact of shame, this finding of the current study might support the need to give temperamental symptoms such as shame at least the same priority as other, more acute symptoms in the treatment of BPD. This is especially important because currently the main effective treatment modalities offered for BPD patients, such as dialectical behavioral therapy (DBT; Linehan, Armstrong, Suarez, Allmon, & Heard, 1991) and mentalization-based therapy (Bateman & Fonagy, 2001), mainly address the acute symptoms of BPD (Zanarini et al., 2007). This need to give shame a higher priority is supported further by the current study's finding of other results of higher shame among BPD patients with comorbid PTSD, which might imply that shame represents a unique and complex experience in BPD that is not addressed as a part of the treatment of BPD.

This study raises clinical implications in regard to treatment offered to patients with BPD. While shame has been overlooked in the study of BPD, it has been found to be a common experience of patients, which also has negative implications for patients' lives (Rüsch, Lieb, et al., 2007; Unoka & Vizin, 2017). It is especially crucial to have a high awareness of patients' experience of shame, because it might not be easy to identify, primarily because it involves avoidant behaviors and can be masked by other emotions, such as anger (Rüsch, Lieb, et al., 2007). Our findings stress the importance and need for formulating intervention programs that will target shame in patients with a BPD diagnosis.

An feature of DBT exposure-based interventions, termed *opposite action*, is another promising part of DBT therapy that has been shown to decrease levels of shame among individuals with BPD (Rizvi & Linehan, 2005). In opposite action, individuals learn to alter an undesirable emotion by recognizing that emotion when it appears, noticing the behaviors that their emotion automatically elicits (called *action tendencies*), but eventually identifying and choosing a behavior that is opposite to those they initially engaged in. The prevention of maladaptive behavioral tendencies by initiating new and opposite ones reinforces the new response pattern while weakening the original emotional response (Linehan, 1993b).

While DBT, in general, has extensive empirical support (Kliem, Kröger, & Kosfelder, 2010), it is its central component, mindfulness, that could be especially effective in reducing shame in BPD. Mindfulness, which is the ability to focus on one's current experiences in the present with acceptance and without judgment (Keng, Smoski, & Robin, 2011), can help in reducing shame in different ways by allowing perceptional change (Shapiro, Carlson, Astin, & Freedman, 2006) because it creates a distance between individuals and their experiences, providing opportunities to reexamine thoughts and feelings and perceive them not as constant or permanent, but as psychological states that change (Keng & Tan, 2017). Mindfulness also has the potential of increasing acceptance of one's own adverse feelings (Baer, 2003). Because mindfulness fosters acceptance of one's feelings rather than criticizing them, it also has the potential to reduce the difficult feelings that people with BPD have toward their own experience of shame (Schoenleber & Berenbaum, 2012) as well as their own views of themselves. According to empirical evidence, mindfulness has been found to successfully decrease shame in individuals with BPD characteristics (Keng et al., 2011) and, considering our findings, it could be helpful to look at shame further within BPD patients.

Limitations

This study has limitations. First, the studies included in this meta-analysis were cross-sectional and thus causality cannot be assumed from the results. Second, the number of studies included in the analysis was relatively small because there is little current literature on the subject. Because the study was a meta-analysis with the comparison value being Cohen's *d*, it did not include studies with just a BPD group, since a healthy control comparison group was required for inclusion in the study. While clinical comparison groups (i.e., patients with a dual diagnosis or other mental health disorders) could have been meaningful in contributing more insight about the prevalence and influence of shame among different diagnoses, the literature was limited in that aspect and thus we chose to focus on BPD alone. Finally, included only studies that used self-report tests or questionnaires because there is currently not one widely used shame paradigm; however, this led to limited inclusion of articles.

Conclusions

In sum, our study provides the first meta-analysis to assess reported shame in BPD patients as compared to healthy controls. Variables such as education level and comorbidity of PTSD were found to have moderate results. The article highlights an important contribution to understanding the experience of BPD patients and to the detection of those who are at a higher risk for experiencing shame. Future studies should continue to evaluate the influence of shame on the lives of individuals with a BPD diagnosis and the ability of different psychotherapeutic approaches to target and reduce shame successfully.

REFERENCES

American Psychiatric Association. (2013). *Diagnostic and statistical manual of mental disorders* (5th ed.). Arlington, VA: American Psychiatric Publishing.

Andrews, B. (1995). Bodily shame as a mediator between abusive experiences and depression. *Journal of Abnormal Psychology, 104*, 277–285.

Andrews, B. (1997). Bodily shame in relation to abuse in childhood and bulimia: A preliminary investigation. *British Journal of Clinical Psychology, 36*, 41–49.

Andrews, B., Brewin, C. R., Rose, S., & Kirk, M. (2000). Predicting PTSD symptoms in victims of violent crime: The role of shame, anger, and childhood abuse. *Journal of Abnormal Psychology, 109*, 69–73.

Andrews, B., Qian, M., & Valentine, J. D. (2002). Predicting depressive symptoms with a new measure of shame: The Experience of Shame Scale. *British Journal of Clinical Psychology, 41*, 29–42.

Baer, R. A. (2003). Mindfulness training as a clinical intervention: A conceptual and empirical review. *Clinical Psychology: Science and Practice, 10*, 125–143.

Bateman, A., & Fonagy, P. (2001). Treatment of borderline personality disorder with psychoanalytically oriented partial hospitalization: An 18-month follow-up. *American Journal of Psychiatry, 158*, 36–42.

Begg, C. B., & Mazumdar, M. (1994). Operating characteristics of a rank correlation test for publication bias. *Biometrics, 50*, 1088–1101.

Bolton, E. E., Mueser, K. T., & Rosenberg, S. D. (2006). Symptom correlates of posttraumatic stress disorder in clients with borderline personality disorder. *Comprehensive Psychiatry, 47*, 357–361.

Borenstein, M., Hedges, L., Higgins, J., & Rothstein, H. (2005). *Comprehensive Meta-Analysis, Version 3*. Biostat.

Brown, M. Z., Comtois, K. A., & Linehan, M. M. (2002). Reasons for suicide attempts and nonsuicidal self-injury in women with borderline personality disorder. *Journal of Abnormal Psychology, 111*, 198–202.

Cameron, A. Y., Erisman, S., & Palm Reed, K. (2020). The relationship among shame, nonsuicidal self-injury, and suicidal behaviors in borderline personality disorder. *Psychological Reports, 123*, 648–659.

Chan, M. A., Hess, G. C., Whelton, W. J., & Yonge, O. J. (2005). A comparison between female psychiatric outpatients with BPD and female university students in terms of trauma, internalized shame and psychiatric symptomatology. *Traumatology, 11*, 23–40.

Cohen, J. (1988). *Statistical power analysis for the behavioral sciences* (2nd ed.). Hillsdale, NJ: Erlbaum.

Dahl, S. (1989). Acute response to rape—A PTSD variant. *Acta Psychiatrica Scandinavica Supplementum, 80*(355), 56–62.

Egger, M., Smith, G., Schneider, M., & Minder, C. (1997). Bias in meta-analysis detected by a simple, graphical test. *BMJ, 315*(7109), 629–634.

Feiring, C., Taska, L., & Lewis, M. (1996). A process model for understanding adaptation to sexual abuse: The role of shame in defining stigmatization. *Child Abuse & Neglect, 20*, 767–782.

Ferguson, T. J., & Crowley, S. L. (1997). Gender differences in the organization of guilt and shame. *Sex Roles, 37*(1–2), 19–44.

Gilbert, P. (1998). What is shame? Some core issues and controversies. In P. Gilbert & B. Andrews (Eds.), *Shame: Interpersonal behavior, psychopathology, and culture* (pp. 3–38). New York, NY: Oxford University Press.

Gratz, K. L., Rosenthal, M. Z., Tull, M. T., Lejuez, C. W., & Gunderson, J. G. (2010). An experimental investigation of emotional reactivity and delayed emotional recovery in borderline personality disorder: The role of shame. *Comprehensive Psychiatry, 51*, 275–285.

Harder, D. W., Cutler, L., & Rockart, L. (1992). Assessment of shame and guilt and their relationships to psychopathology. *Journal of Personality Assessment, 59*, 584–604.

Harvey, O. J., Gore, E. J., Frank, H., & Batres, A. R. (1997). Relationship of shame and guilt to gender and parenting practices. *Personality and Individual Differences, 23*, 135–146.

Hasson-Ohayon, I., Ehrlich-Ben Or, S., Vahab, K., Amiaz, R., Weiser, M., & Roe, D. (2012). Insight into mental illness and self-stigma: The mediating role of shame proneness. *Psychiatry Research, 200*(2–3), 802–806.

Hedges, L. V., & Olkin, I. (1985). *Statistical methods for meta-analysis*. Orlando, FL: Academic Press.

Herman, J. L. (1992). *Trauma and recovery*. New York, NY: Basic Books.

Jacob, G. A., Hellstern, K., Ower, N., Pillmann, M., Scheel, C. N., Rüsch, N., & Lieb, K. (2009). Emotional reactions to standardized stimuli in women with borderline personality disorder: Stronger negative affect, but no differences in reactivity. *Journal of Nervous and Mental Disease, 197*, 808–815.

Karan, E., Niesten, I. J. M., Frankenburg, F. R., Fitzmaurice, G. M., & Zanarini, M. C. (2014). The 16-year course of shame and its risk factors in patients with borderline personality disorder: Course of shame and its risk factors in BPD. *Personality and Mental Health, 8*, 169–177.

Keng, S. L., Smoski, M. J., & Robins, C. J. (2011). Effects of mindfulness on psychological health: A review of empirical studies. *Clinical Psychology Review, 31*, 1041–1056.

Keng, S. L., & Tan, J. X. (2017). Effects of brief mindful breathing and loving-kindness meditation on shame and social problem solving abilities among individuals with high borderline personality traits. *Behaviour Research and Therapy, 97*, 43–51.

Kernberg, O. (1984). *Object relations theory and clinical psychoanalysis*. New York, NY: Aronson.

Kliem, S., Kröger, C., & Kosfelder, J. (2010). Dialectical behavior therapy for borderline personality disorder: A meta-analysis using mixed-effects modeling. *Journal of Consulting and Clinical Psychology, 78*, 936–951.

Lester, D. (1997). The role of shame in suicide. *Suicide & Life-Threatening Behavior, 27*, 352–361.

Lewis, H. B. (1971). Shame and guilt in neurosis. *Psychoanalytic Review, 58*, 419–438.

Lieb, K., Zanarini, M. C., Schmahl, C., Linehan, M. M., & Bohus, M. (2004). Borderline personality disorder. *Lancet, 364*(9432), 453–461.

Linehan, M. M. (1993a). *Cognitive behavioral treatment of borderline personality disorder*. New York, NY: Guilford Press.

Linehan, M. M. (1993b). *Skills training manual for treating borderline personality disorder*. New York, NY: Guilford Press.

Linehan, M. M., Armstrong, H. E., Suarez, A., Allmon, D., & Heard, H. L. (1991). Cognitive-behavioral treatment of chronically parasuicidal borderline patients. *Archives of General Psychiatry, 48*, 1060–1064.

Mills, R. S. L. (2005). Taking stock of the developmental literature on shame. *Developmental Review, 25*, 26–63.

Nathanson, D. L. (1994). Shame, compassion, and the "borderline" personality. *Psychiatric Clinics of North America, 17*, 785–810.

Orth, U., Robins, R. W., & Soto, C. J. (2010). Tracking the trajectory of shame, guilt, and pride across the life span. *Journal of Personality and Social Psychology, 99*, 1061–1071.

Paris, J., Brown, R., & Nowlis, D. (1987). Long-term follow-up of borderline patients in a general hospital. *Comprehensive Psychiatry, 28*, 530–535.

Pinto-Gouveia, J., & Matos, M. (2011). Can shame memories become a key to identity? The centrality of shame memories predicts psychopathology. *Applied Cognitive Psychology, 25*, 281–290.

Ritter, K., Vater, A., Rüsch, N., Schröder-Abé, M., Schütz, A., Fydrich, T., ,... Roepke, S. (2014). Shame in patients with narcissistic personality disorder. *Psychiatry Research, 215*, 429–437.

Rizvi, S. L., & Linehan, M. M. (2005). The treatment of maladaptive shame in borderline personality disorder: A pilot study of "opposite action." *Cognitive and Behavioral Practice, 12*, 437–447.

Roberts, B. W., & Damian, R. I. (2019). The principles of personality trait development and their relation to psychopathology. In D. B. Samuel & D. R. Lynam (Eds.), *Using basic personality research to inform personality pathology* (pp. 153–168). New York, NY: Oxford University Press.

Roberts, B. W., Wood, D., & Caspi, A. (2008). The development of personality traits in adulthood. In O. John, R. Robins, & L. Pervin (Eds.), *Handbook of personality: Theory and research* (pp. 375–398). New York, NY: Guilford Press.

Rüsch, N., Corrigan, P. W., Bohus, M., Kühler, T., Jacob, G. A., & Lieb, K. (2007). The impact of posttraumatic stress disorder on dysfunctional implicit and explicit emotions among women with borderline personality disorder. *Journal of Nervous and Mental Disease, 195*, 537–539.

Rüsch, N., Lieb, K., Göttler, I., Hermann, C., Schramm, E., Richter, H., ,... Bohus, M. (2007). Shame and implicit self-concept in women with borderline personality disorder. *American Journal of Psychiatry, 164*, 500–508.

Saraiya, T., & Lopez-Castro, T. (2016). Ashamed and afraid: A scoping review of the role of shame in post-traumatic stress disorder (PTSD). *Journal of Clinical Medicine, 5*(11), 94.

Scheel, C. N., Bender, C., Tuschen-Caffier, B., Brodführer, A., Matthies, S., Hermann, C., ... Jacob, G. A. (2014). Do patients with different mental disorders show specific aspects of shame? *Psychiatry Research, 220*(1–2), 490–495.

Schoenleber, M., & Berenbaum, H. (2012). Aversion and proneness to shame in self and informant reported personality disorder symptoms. *Personality Disorders, 3*, 294–304.

Shapiro, S. L., Carlson, L. E., Astin, J. A., & Freedman, B. (2006). Mechanisms of mindfulness. *Journal of Clinical Psychology, 62*, 373–386.

Sippel, L. M., & Marshall, A. D. (2011). Posttraumatic stress disorder symptoms, intimate partner violence perpetration, and the mediating role of shame processing bias. *Journal of Anxiety Disorders, 25*, 903–910.

Stein, M. B., & Kean, Y. M. (2000). Disability and quality of life in social phobia: Epidemiologic findings. *American Journal of Psychiatry, 157*, 1606–1613.

Stevenson, J., Meares, R., & Comerford, A. (2003). Diminished impulsivity in older patients with borderline personality disorder. *American Journal of Psychiatry, 160*, 165–166.

Stone, M. (2001). Natural history and long-term outcome. In W. Livesley (Ed.), *Handbook of personality disorders: Theory, research, and treatment* (pp. 259–273). New York, NY: Guilford Press.

Tangney, J. P., Miller, R. S., Flicker, L., & Barlow, D. H. (1996). Are shame, guilt, and embarrassment distinct emotions? *Journal of Personality and Social Psychology, 70*, 1256–1269.

Tangney, J. P., Stuewig, J., & Mashek, D. J. (2007). Moral emotions and moral behavior. *Annual Review of Psychology, 58*, 345–372.

Tomkins, S. (1963). *Affect imagery consciousness: Volume II: The negative affects*. New York, NY: Springer Publishing Company.

Tracy, J. L., & Matsumoto, D. (2008). The spontaneous expression of pride and shame: Evidence for biologically innate nonverbal displays. *Proceedings of the National Academy of Sciences of the United States of America, 105*(33), 11655–11660.

Unoka, Z., & Vizin, G. (2017). To see in a mirror dimly. The looking glass self is self-shaming in borderline personality disorder. *Psychiatry Research, 258*, 322–329.

Vizin, G., Urbán, R., & Unoka, Z. (2016). Shame, trauma, temperament and psychopathology: Construct validity of the Experience of Shame Scale. *Psychiatry Research, 246*, 62–69.

Wilson, J. P., Drozdek, B., & Turkovic, S. (2006). Posttraumatic shame and guilt. *Trauma, Violence & Abuse, 7*, 122–141.

Wright, F., & O'Leary, J. (1989). Shame, guilt, narcissism, and depression: Correlates and sex differences. *Psychoanalytic Psychology, 6*, 217–230.

Young, J. E., Klosko, J. S., & Weishaar, M. E. (2003). *Schema therapy: A practitioner's guide*. New York, NY: Guilford Press.

Zanarini, M. C., Frankenburg, F. R., Reich, D. B., Silk, K. R., Hudson, J. I., & McSweeney, L. B. (2007). The subsyndromal phenomenology of borderline personality disorder: A 10-year follow-up study. *American Journal of Psychiatry, 164*, 929–935.

Zanarini, M. C., Yong, L., Frankenburg, F. R., Hennen, J., Reich, D. B., Marino, M. F., & Vujanovic, A. A. (2002). Severity of reported childhood sexual abuse and its relationship to severity of borderline psychopathology and psychosocial impairment among borderline inpatients. *Journal of Nervous and Mental Disease, 190*, 381–387.

www.ingramcontent.com/pod-product-compliance
Ingram Content Group UK Ltd.
Pitfield, Milton Keynes, MK11 3LW, UK
UKHW052129260125
454224UK00006B/24